# PANDEMIC IN POTOSÍ

# PANDEMIC IN POTOSÍ

Fear, Loathing, and Public Piety in a Colonial Mining Metropolis

**Kris Lane**

The Pennsylvania State University Press
University Park, Pennsylvania

*Frontispiece* Saint Rose of Lima, Madrid, 1711. Courtesy of the John Carter Brown Library at Brown University, Providence, RI.

Library of Congress Cataloging-in-Publication Data

Names: Lane, Kris E., 1967– author.
Title: Pandemic in Potosí : fear, loathing, and public piety in a colonial mining metropolis / Kris Lane.
Other titles: Latin American originals ; 18.
Description: University Park, Pennsylvania : The Pennsylvania State University Press, [2021] | Series: Latin American originals ; 18 | Includes bibliographical references and index.
Summary: "Narrative accounts, translated into English, of a pandemic that swept across South America between 1717 and 1722, devastating the cities of Buenos Aires, Córdoba, Potosí, Arequipa, and Cuzco as well as many smaller towns"—Provided by publisher.
Identifiers: LCCN 2021037443 | ISBN 9780271091983 (paperback)
Subjects: LCSH: Epidemics—Bolivia—Potosí—History—18th century—Sources. | Epidemics—South America—History—18th century—Sources. | LCGFT: Personal narratives.
Classification: LCC RA650.55.B6 L36 2021 | DDC 614.40984/14—dc23
LC record available at https://lccn.loc.gov/2021037443

*Paradoxical as it may sound, the lesson of history is that all too often people find it easier to manip-ulate the facts to fit their theories than to adapt their theories to the facts observed.*

—Carlo Cipolla, *Fighting the Plague in Seventeenth-Century Italy*

CONTENTS

# ILLUSTRATIONS

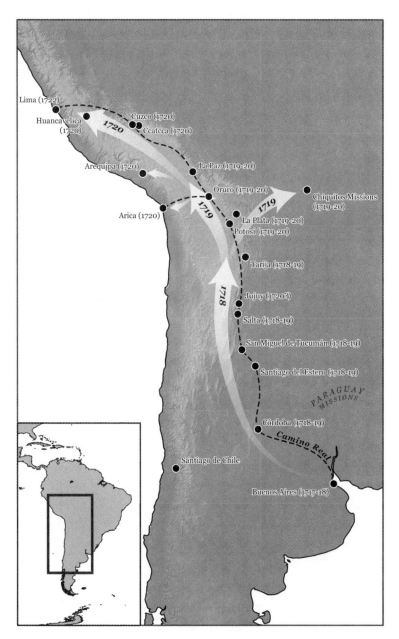

MAP 1. Map of South America, showing the trajectory of the 1717–22 pandemic.

Latin American Originals (LAO) is a series of primary-source texts on colonial Latin America. LAO volumes are accessible editions of texts translated from more than seven European and Indigenous American languages into English—most of them for the very first time. Of the eighteen volumes now in print, half illuminate aspects of the Spanish invasions in the Americas during the long century of 1494–1614. The others take the series in varied and exciting directions, from the forging of new Christianities to medical science to dealings with death—to which the present volume makes a stirring contribution.

Taken in the chronological order of their primary texts, *Of Cannibals and Kings* (LAO 7) comes first. It presents the earliest written attempts to describe Indigenous American cultures, offering striking insight into how Europeans struggled from the very start to conceive a "New World." *The Native Conquistador* (LAO 10) tells the story of the (in)famous Spanish Conquest expeditions into Mexico and Central America from 1519 to 1524—but from the startlingly different perspective of a royal Indigenous dynasty, as told by the great-great-grandson of the alternative leading protagonist.

Next, chronologically, are LAOs 2, 1, then 9. *Invading Guatemala* shows how reading multiple accounts of conquest wars (in this case, Spanish, Nahua, and Maya versions of the Guatemalan conflict of the 1520s) can explode established narratives and suggest a more complex and revealing conquest story. *Invading Colombia* challenges us to view the difficult Spanish invasion of Colombia in the 1530s as more representative of conquest campaigns than the better-known assaults on the Aztec and Inca Empires. It complements *The Improbable Conquest*, which presents letters written between 1537 and 1556 by Spaniards struggling—with a persistence that is improbable indeed—to plant a colony along the hopefully named Río de la Plata.

Volume 12 adds intriguingly to that trio. *Contesting Conquest* offers new perspectives on Nueva Galicia's understudied early history. Indigenous witnesses and informants, their voices deftly identified, selected, and presented, guide us through the grim, messy tale of repeated efforts at conquest and colonization from the late 1520s through 1545.

Continuing chronologically, LAOs 11, 3, 4, and 16 all explore aspects of the aftermath and legacy of the invasion era. *The History of the New World* offers the first English translation since 1847 of part of a 1565 Italian book that, in its day, was a best seller in five languages. The merchant-adventurer Girolamo Benzoni mixed sharp observations and sympathy for Indigenous peoples with imaginary tales and wild history, influencing generations of early modern readers and challenging modern readers to sort out fact from fable. *The Conquest on Trial* features a fictional Indigenous embassy filing a complaint in a court in Spain—the Court of Death. The first theatrical examination of the conquest published in Spain, it effectively condensed contemporary debates on colonization into one dramatic package. It contrasts well with *Defending the Conquest*, which presents a spirited, ill-humored, and polemic apologia for the Spanish Conquest, written in 1613 by a veteran conquistador. *Indigenous Life After the Conquest* presents the papers of a Nahua family, showing how family members navigated the gradual changes and challenges that swept central Mexico in the century after the dramatic upheaval of invasion and conquest. Through Indigenous eyes, we see how a new order was built, contested, shaped, and reconfigured by Nahuas themselves.

LAO 16 dovetails in many ways with volumes 13, 6, 5, and 8—which explore aspects of Spanish efforts to implant Christianity in the Americas. In order, *To Heaven or to Hell* leads the pack, presenting the first complete English translation of a book by Bartolomé de Las Casas. Originally published in 1552, his *Confessionary for Confessors*—soon overshadowed by his famous *Very Brief Account of the Destruction of the Indies*—was initially just as controversial; conquistadors and other Spaniards were outraged by its demand that they themselves be effectively made subject to the so-called spiritual conquest.

*Gods of the Andes* presents the first English edition of a 1594 manuscript describing Inca religion and the campaign to convert

Indigenous Andeans. Its Jesuit author is surprisingly sympathetic to preconquest beliefs and practices, viewing them as preparing Andeans for the arrival of the new faith. *Forgotten Franciscans* casts new light on conversion campaigns and the conflictive cultural world of the Inquisition in sixteenth-century Mexico. Both LAO 6 and 5 expose wildly divergent views within the Spanish American church on Indigenous religions and how to replace them with Christianity. Complementing those two volumes by revealing the Indigenous side to the same process, *Translated Christianities* presents religious texts translated from Nahuatl and Yucatec Maya. Designed to proselytize and ensure the piety of Indigenous parishioners, these texts show how such efforts actually contributed to the development of local Christianities.

LAOs 17 and 14 take the series into the seventeenth century. *An Irish Rebel in New Spain* casts a sharp eye on the far-reaching intrigues of colonial and inquisitorial politics. William Lamport, aka the Irish Zorro, rose through colonial Mexican society only to lose his life in the clutches of the Holy Office. LAO 17 explores his dramatic life, theological philosophies, and provocative writings to shed light on the cruel whimsy of (mis)fortune in a time of upheaval and instability in Spanish America. Through the "Journal and History" of a Dutch expedition to Chile, LAO 14 extends the series into yet another region of the Americas; *To the Shores of Chile* opens up a new perspective on European-Indigenous interaction, colonization, and global competition in the age of empire.

Taken chronologically, LAOs 18 and 15 take the series into the eighteenth century—and continue its move in bold new directions. This latest addition to the series, *Pandemic in Potosí*, presents in translation a 1719 account of the great plague that devastated the Andean mining metropolis, augmenting the suffering of a population already burdened by dramatic declines in silver production. Yet Potosí's inhabitants found ways to adapt and survive amid a pandemic that took the lives of one in three of them. As well as echoing events in our own time, LAO 18 weaves together many of the themes explored in other volumes in the series—from sin and salvation to science and medicine. That takes us both chronologically and thematically to LAO 15, which uses an eighteenth-century Guatemalan case study to explore the fascinating intersections between faith and science in the early modern world. *Baptism Through Incision* presents an eye-opening 1786 treatise on performing cesareans on pregnant women at the moment of their death, contributing to LAO series themes such as empire, salvation, the female body, and knowledge as a battleground. The source texts in LAO volumes are colonial-era rare books or archival documents, written in European or Indigenous languages. LAO authors are historians, anthropologists, art historians, geographers, and scholars of literature who have developed a specialized knowledge that allows them to locate, translate, and present these texts in a way that contributes to scholars' understanding of the period, while also making them readable for students and nonspecialists. World-renowned scholar of many aspects of the history of early Latin America, Kris Lane is also a veteran LAO author, so his deft and engaging style now graces this series twice.

—Matthew Restall

Disease epidemics have a way of concentrating the mind and testing human capacities. How did past societies cope with pandemics or global pathogens spread when vaccinations and other modern medical interventions were unavailable, even unthinkable? This collection of primary sources from eighteenth-century South America spotlights local reactions to a previously unknown ailment. In 1719 a pandemic ravaged the silver-mining city of Potosí, in present-day Bolivia, after devastating Buenos Aires and Córdoba, Argentina. Possibly introduced via the transatlantic slave trade, the pathogen went on to cripple Cuzco and Arequipa, Peru, decimating many smaller, mostly Indigenous towns along the way. In all, the disease killed hundreds of thousands and displaced many more.

If early modern medical therapies were of limited use against virulent pathogens, what were the options? Was social distancing practiced, or masking? Generally no, but none sat idly by as the pandemic raged. The Andes region of South America was deeply Roman Catholic by this time, and, as such, believers put their trust in Jesus Christ, Mary, and the saints as intercessors before God. Catholic priests, self-appointed frontline workers of their day, according to observers, cared for the sick and "cured souls." Priests urged parishioners to respond to the health crisis with religious processions and other acts of collective piety. Personal pleas for forgiveness followed. A sinner's best hope when struck by "contagion" was a good death, making peace with family, neighbors, and God before expiring.

Thankfully for us, the Gran Peste that swept the Andes between 1717 and 1722 left a documentary trail. The sources collected and translated here reveal the alarm and drama that accompanied an early modern American pandemic, along with the search for answers (and culprits). There is evidence, too, of an emerging med-ical science rooted in Enlightenment principles, and, although early eighteenth-century theories of disease causation and prescribed therapies may seem ludicrous today, sources point to experimentation to help limit suffering. The pandemic provoked conflict between established faith and newfangled science.

In what may have been a global coincidence, an equally deadly pathogen struck Marseille and parts of southern France in 1720. Marseille's experience merits brief comparison, in part because it coincided with the Andean pandemic but also because conflicting reactions to it illuminate common stress points, some found in more recent pandemics. These include (1) calls for isolationism and self-sufficiency versus openness and global interdependency; (2) denunciations of opportunism, debauchery, and carelessness amid chaos and death versus praise for civic duty, self-sacrifice, and moral integrity; (3) class solidarity versus antagonism or division; (4) the promotion of novel medical and public health interventions versus quack remedies or false palliatives; and (5) the search for cosmic causes and meaning versus more secular views of nature and the limitations of human knowledge. Alert readers will spot many more.

## ACKNOWLEDGMENTS

I thank Alix Rivière for her fluid translations from the French and Michael Brumbaugh for his nonpareil Latin. Tim Johnson and an anonymous reader deciphered Bartolomé Arzáns's trickier phrasings. I am especially grateful to Prof. Gabriela Ramos for kindly sharing her vital work on this dark episode, publication of which was delayed by the Great Pandemic of 2020–21. Thanks also go to Alex Borucki, Cindy Ermus, Emily Floyd, David Garrett, Kenneth Mills, Elise Mitchell, Fabrício Prado, Federico Sartori, Sinclair Thomson, Lisa Voigt, Chuck Walker, Adam Warren, and Farren Yero for essential comments and suggestions. Tulane University's Latin American Library staff shared rare materials amid quarantine. Thanks also go to Edith Sandler of the Library of Congress Manuscript Division for photographing the Herrera y Loyzaga manuscript amid lockdown and to Raúl Montero Quispe, who photographed the sobering "pandemic mural" in Ccatcca, Peru. Gracias also to Geoff Wallace for the excellent map. Huge thanks go to Ellie Goodman and Maddie Caso of Penn State University Press, to copyeditor Susan Silver, and to the anonymous readers who reminded me to add student goggles to my face mask. And, finally, I thank Matthew Restall for goading me to turn a "sick" teaching module into a book.

# Introduction

In the year 1719 a deadly and highly contagious disease visited a fading silver-mining metropolis known as the Imperial Villa of Potosí, located high in the Andes Mountains of south-central Bolivia—or so we are told by town chronicler Bartolomé Arzáns de Orsúa y Vela, an eyewitness and survivor. Arzáns, as he is known to scholars and townsfolk, composed his million-word *History of the Imperial Villa of Potosí* between 1705 and 1736, until death stilled his pen.[1] The great 1719 plague, or *peste*, as Arzáns and others called it, was a pivotal event he narrated at length, in part because he lived through it but also because it was shot through with cosmic significance.

Following the punishments of the seventeenth century, the great 1719 peste came as a surprise in the middle of Arzáns's composition, a "fourth strike." The great pandemic, which devastated much of Spanish Peru, at that time including Argentina, Paraguay, Bolivia, and Chile, hit Potosí just as the Silver City was at its lowest point, with less than half the population of a century before. Silver production had all but collapsed after a modest revival in the 1690s, when worked-out mines flooded both in Potosí and in its many satellite camps. Throughout the Andes, Quechua- and Aymara-speaking Indigenous communities struggled to recover from centuries of forced labor, disease, and displacement.

Yet amid this decadence a new, semilegal trade opened up with foreigners, first the French and then the British, during and after the War of the Spanish Succession (1702–13), cause for hope in Potosí's

---

1. Arzáns de Orsúa y Vela, *Historia*.

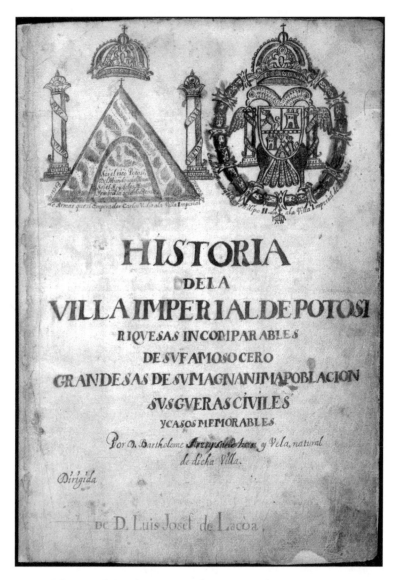

FIG. 1. Title page of Bartolomé Arzáns de Orsúa y Vela's manuscript *Historia de la Villa Imperial de Potosí*. Courtesy of the John Hay Library at Brown University, Providence, RI.

business community. Increased trade, or consumption, they believed, would stimulate mining investment. Foreign penetration was two-pronged. The brutal traffic in enslaved Africans via Buenos Aires grew as Spain's former enemies formed joint-stock companies, as did imports of luxury textiles via French merchants, mostly on the Pacific coast.[2] Some *potosinos* were hopeful that newly arrived foreign merchants, despite their heretical tendencies, would spur revival. And the influx of enslaved Africans, they believed, would offset Indigenous population decline, renovating the workforce. Arzáns, a tireless moralist, was less optimistic. He saw foreign trade stimulating contraband, tax evasion, and worse.

The years around 1719 were fraught. Potosí's registered silver production had dropped from a high of nearly 1.8 million kilograms in the 1590s to under 1 million kilograms in the 1650s.[3] Decline steepened such that in the first decade of the eighteenth century, the king taxed only 395,190 kilograms of silver. Output kept dropping: 347,500 kilograms in the 1710s and 325,870 kilograms in the 1720s—roughly one-sixth of what it had been at its height. Amid decline, the new Bourbon king, Philip V, outlawed the infamous *mita* labor draft. Mine labor would be much more costly as a result, yet, as Arzáns notes near the end of the 1719–20 narrative, Potosí's industrial elite, owners of mines and refineries, convinced Peru's viceroy to delay implementing the ban until the king could be persuaded to change his mind.

Yet few, including Arzáns, could deny that the mita, formalized in 1572, was massively deadly and disruptive to native Andean populations throughout present-day Bolivia and Peru.[4] It had all but hollowed out great expanses of the central Andes.[5] Even so, Andeans proved adaptive, finding ways to survive and occasionally thrive despite the demands of the mita and other hardships. Amazingly, a growing number of Indigenous men and women found modest success in the silver industry, including in the Rich Hill, or Cerro Rico, itself.

2. See the circa 1712 map for South Sea Company investors with a Cerro Rico inset: Moll, Lens, and Vertue, "This Map of South America."
3. TePaske, *New World*, 190–91. Annual registered silver production dropped in 1719 and 1720, recovering in 1728 (189).
4. Lane, *Potosí*, 142–57.
5. Dell, "Persistent Effects."

As Enrique Tandeter and Rossana Barragán have shown, the practice of *kajcheo*, or removing high-grade ore when the mines were officially closed, made up a significant share of total Potosí silver production in the early eighteenth century.[6] The practice of high grading pitted the old industrialists against native Andean miners, many of them by this time wageworkers. Small-scale refiners, some of them women, also flourished, further eroding the mill owners' power.

Arzáns sometimes pauses to comment on long-term trends, but his annalistic *History* has a more event-rich and immediate flavor. For the moralizing town chronicler, the years after 1700 were marred by the same sins that had provoked divine punishment in the past. Each year brought renewed disputes between grasping Crown officials and greedy local elites, torrid love affairs and their violent consequences, cave-ins and other mine disasters, cold-blooded murders, jail breaks, celestial disturbances, disease outbreaks, and climatic variations, occasionally broken up by the arrival of good or bad news from Madrid or Rome, prompting a massive, days-long festival or requiem.

The year 1702, for example, witnessed riots sparked by a high-profile murder, followed by celebrations for the canonization of Saint John of God. In 1705 the Virgin Mary saved an Indigenous miner's life, but this was offset by public brawls and a minor epidemic. In 1707 rancor and division continued as the king banned French clothing. This edict and a forbidden love affair prompted protests, cut short by another pathogen. Good news came a few years later regarding Philip V's contested succession, but in 1712 drought struck, idling the city's hydraulic silver refineries. In 1713 Potosí hosted the new archbishop of La Plata, Fray Diego Morcillo Rubio de Auñón, and in 1716 Archbishop Morcillo was unexpectedly named viceroy of Peru in lieu of a replacement from Madrid, making him the first viceroy to visit Potosí since Francisco de Toledo back in the 1570s. The Imperial Villa gave Morcillo the royal treatment.

According to Arzáns, who cannot help sermonizing on greed, pride, envy, and other sins midstory, the archbishop-viceroy entered Potosí by way of an elaborate triumphal arch at three in the

---

6. Tandeter, *Coercion and Market*; Barragán, "Working Silver"; Barragán, "Ladrones."

afternoon on April 25, 1716.[7] There would follow nearly two weeks
of nonstop feasts, plays, equestrian games, bullfights, masquerades,
musical performances, and ritual processions and dedications, the
likes of which Potosí had not experienced (much less financed) for
many decades. Arzáns says municipal officials viewed the festivities
as a necessary investment.

As he does in describing the largest religious processions sent out
to halt the great 1719 pandemic, Arzáns spares no detail in describing how his hometown welcomed quasi royalty. Every architectural
element, every flower, every candle, and every fabric type, texture,
and color are listed. If we close our eyes, we can almost see the totter-
ing triumphal arches; the resplendent baroque facades; the liveried,
marching musketeers; and the hundreds of prominent women and
their servants looking down on the parade from their balconies,
with paintings and tapestries hung out to enhance the visual feast.
Fortunately, Potosí's most famous painter, Melchor Pérez Holguín,
bore witness to this spectacle, and his largest surviving canvas depicts
the entrance of the archbishop-viceroy to the Imperial Villa almost as
Arzáns describes it.

Here is Arzáns on the women of Potosí as they look down on the
dignitary:

> With mace and pallium His Excellency began to walk through
> those streets; springtime of the fairer sex, as they filled the
> balconies, windows, and grandstands made for the purpose, so
> many illustrious matrons, so many honest damsels, so many
> celebrated ladies, all gallant and richly adorned, and on no other
> occasion had one seen brought together for the augmentation
> of the beauty of their faces so many jewels, so many precious
> stones, nor such riches in pearls, so gracious and smiling were
> they, giving a thousand well wishes to His Excellency, stealing
> the task from Flora, all beauty from Diana, and indeed the very
> eyes of those who gazed upon them.[8]

For an author given to railing against the mortal dangers of female
beauty, Arzáns seems transported by this spectacular occasion. Yet he

7. Arzáns de Orsúa y Vela, *Historia*, 3:47–53.
8. Ibid., 3:48.

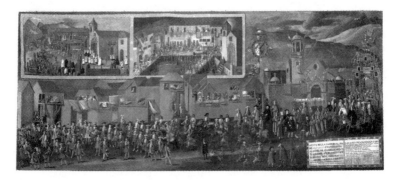

FIG. 2. Melchor Pérez Holguín's *Entrada del Arzobispo-Virrey Morcillo en la Villa Imperial de Potosí*. Courtesy of Museo de América, Madrid, Spain.

could not help but add, after a bit more hyperbole, that this charming, feminine facade hid rotten foundations and sinister urges. First, he grumbled, the city had wasted a fortune on gaudy French fashions, and, second, Potosí's extraordinary array of beautiful women of all classes and nationalities, when combined with the city's less salutary and equally diverse masculine energies, were a recipe for disaster, or rather "eternal perdition."[9]

Yet even Arzáns could not help but gloat at how the procession proved that, even in decline, the Imperial Villa could put on a world-class show. After eight days of partying, His Eminence gave the following statement: "You have given me too much, Potosí. I shall remember your liberality. And now I don't wish to linger any longer so as to not bother you further."[10] Loaded with gifts (or bribes), including nearly a ton of untaxed silver, if we may trust Arzáns, Morcillo left the town for the long trip to Lima. Barely outside Potosí city limits, news arrived that the "real" viceroy, the prince of Santo Buono, a fashionably coiffed Neapolitan, was about to reach Lima via Panama. The slowness of transoceanic communication had cost the city dearly, and Arzáns says the news left *potosinos* as despondent as they were bankrupt. Morcillo wisely skirted Potosí on his way back to La Plata.

9. Ibid.
10. Ibid., 3:49.

In 1717 contraband trade disputes resurged amid good news regarding the Holy Roman emperor's military successes in Hungary plus the beatification of two Jesuits. Potosí's silver refiners were stunned to hear that the king had after all abolished the mita, an apparent victory for native Andeans. Shrill appeals were promptly drafted. The year 1718 continued with Crown crackdowns on contraband trade via Buenos Aires and ended with the arrival of a new governor, or *corregidor*, just in time for the Gran Peste.

Fortunately, we have a visitor's sketch of Potosí (fig. 3) on the eve of pandemic. A government official who later became head of the district court, José Cipriano Herrera y Loyzaga, reached Potosí on December 27, 1717, from Buenos Aires, having left on September 8. He noted the following: "[Potosí] has a very great number of Indians, as the Spaniards inhabit only the principal blocks around the square, with their main parish church, whereas the Indians have thirteen [parishes], all of them meticulous and clean in their devotion to the divine cult, and ordinarily some six thousand or seven thousand mita Indians come to town each year."[11]

This brief overview of Arzáns's *History* for the years leading up to the 1719–20 pandemic suggests continuity or, rather, baroque declension: things were bad and getting worse, and sickness often came to town. Reversals of fortune brightened the outlook from time to time, occasion for monumental parties. Potosí was not the great city it had once been, yet this did not prevent French and English merchants, the king of Spain, an interim viceroy, and many others, including Arzáns himself, from believing revival was but one lucky strike away. The great pandemic crushed these hopes. It would not be until after 1750 that Potosí's Indigenous population rebounded and that new policies revived the silver-mining industry just in time for another blow: the wars of independence.

---

11. Herrera y Loyzaga, "Viaje," quote on 143. The original manuscript is in the US Library of Congress, call number S.A. Ac.7.

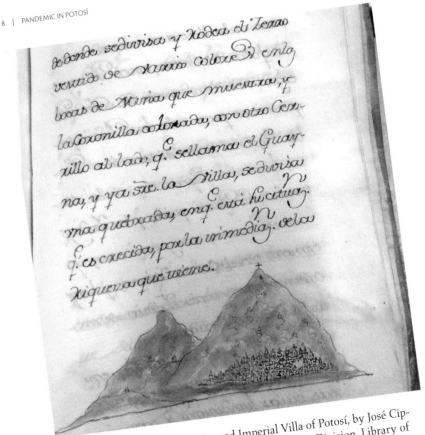

FIG. 3. A sketch of the Cerro Rico and Imperial Villa of Potosí, by José Cipriano Herrera y Loyzaga. Courtesy of the Manuscript Division, Library of Congress, Washington, DC.

## The 1717–22 Pandemic in Greater Peru

Historians of medicine have long noted that the frightfully deadly disease that struck Potosí in 1719 was part of a continental if not pan-Atlantic pandemic that began around 1717 and faded in 1722.[12] Arzáns himself claimed that the illness devastated Buenos Aires and its hinterland, Jesuit missions in Paraguay, the inland cities of Córdoba and Salta, and even Santiago de Chile (which appears to have been spared). A late eighteenth-century source suggests the pandemic was triggered by the landing of a single "death ship," the *French Lion*, somewhere "on the coasts of South America."[13] Fanciful as this may sound, it may not be wrong.

As Susana Frías and María Inés Montserrat have shown, the Gran Peste may have arrived with English slave traders, as Arzáns and other narrators claimed.[14] Using town council records and letters, including annual Jesuit reports and governors' dispatches, Frías and Montserrat found reports of "putrid fevers" in Buenos Aires by July 1717, heart of the Southern Hemisphere winter and in the midst of a multiyear drought. Town council records refer to two English slave ships in port at this time, one awaiting a return cargo of hides (and contraband Potosí silver) and the other quarantined after reports of smallpox on board.[15]

The online Trans-Atlantic Slave Trade Database lists a number of slave ships calling at Buenos Aires between 1716 and 1719, all but

12. Dobyns, "Outline of Andean Epidemic History." Dobyns uses Esquivel on Cuzco but not Arzáns on Potosí, as the *Historia* was unavailable before 1965 (511–15). Dobyns also cites Unanue but not Bottoni. His main source was Lastres, *Medicina en el virreinato*. Dobyns suspected a plague, since pack animals died, but suggested the Gran Peste was epidemic typhus, rife in northwest Europe in the summer of 1718–19 (514). Dobyns confuses Indian "complexion" with skin type on page 514, when *complexión caliente* in the source approximates "hot constitution."
    13. The best take on the Gran Peste is by Ramos, *Cuerpo en palabras*, 119–65. Ramos solves the *French Lion* mystery and suggests the possibility of a hemorrhagic fever originating in Buenos Aires's pampas (home of arenavirus variants).
    14. Frías and Montserrat, "Pestes y muerte"; Arzáns de Orsúa y Vela, *Historia*, 3:77.
    15. Biedma, *Acuerdos del extinguido cabildo*, 426, 474–75, 479, 524, 533–34, 587, 600, 614–16. Elise Mitchell (email message to the author, August 8, 2020) notes that the slave ship *Indian Queen* was quarantined from November to December 1715 (mentioned in the town council minutes as *La Reyna de la India*). See Biedma, *Acuerdos del extinguido cabildo*, 241–42, 254–57. Its voyage was atypical, having left Jamaica for Buenos Aires after stopping in Portobelo (Panama).

one of them English (see table 1).[16] For some idea of what horrors these bland names, dates, and numbers hide, one need only click the ship name for a voyage to piece together a narrative from the "Full Detail." For example, the misnamed ship *Hope*, with a crew of 24, captained by Walter Cronker, left London on August 19, 1715. Flagged for the South Sea Company, the *Hope* reached Cabinda near the mouth of the Zaire River to embark enslaved Africans on January 26, 1716. After several months' cruising, Cronker purchased 369 individuals, his crew packing them into the hold of the tiny, 120-ton ship. By the time the *Hope* reached Buenos Aires in December 1716, only 188 captives were disembarked. The "Full Detail" ends, noting that this represents a mortality rate of 49.1 percent.

More accursed voyages followed. The 350-ton company ship *George*, captained by William Malthus, with a crew of 45, left London on May 26, 1716, reaching Loango, north of Cabinda, later that year. Malthus and his men eventually embarked 594 captives after a long layover. By the time the *George*, presumably named for Britain's new king, dropped anchor at Buenos Aires on July 10, 1717, she carried only 245 living captives, of whom all but 2 were disembarked.

The *George* was likely the quarantined ship mentioned in the Buenos Aires town council minutes and later referred to by Jesuits in the interior. According to the Slave Trade Database, the voyage of the *George* killed 351 captive Africans in the Middle Passage, a jaw-dropping 59 percent mortality rate. Presumably, the *George*

---

16. See Trans-Atlantic Slave Trade Database. Some ships appear in English or French official records, others in Spanish or local records. Compare with Palmer, *Human Cargoes*, 120. See also Borucki, "From Asiento to Spanish Networks," 181–85. As Borucki shows, the Slave Trade Database seems reliable for these years, but some ships brought enslaved Africans illegally to Buenos Aires via the Portuguese enclave of Colônia do Sacramento. As Fabrício Prado has shown, Colônia had just been refounded in late 1716 by Rio-based Portuguese merchants when the peste hit Buenos Aires, followed by a 1718–19 famine. In a letter dated January 6, 1719, Colônia's governor lamented mass desertion, as soldiers and settlers foraged for "wild herbs and fennel," now living "without diet" (i.e., not eating the foods needed to maintain humoral balance and thus disease resistance). He also requested drugs from Rio. See Arquivo Histórico Ultramarino, Lisbon, Conselho Ultramarino, Brasil, Nova Colônia do Sacramento, AHU_ACL_CU_012, Cx.1, D.43. Special thanks to Fabrício Prado for this material. See also Prado, *Anglo-Portuguese Cooperation*. Prado kindly checked registries for Rio de Janeiro Resgate documents in the AHU and found "no references to famine, plague, or even quarantined ships [at the port of Rio] between 1718 and 1720" (email message to the author, April 8, 2020).

Table 1 Registered slave ships landing at Buenos Aires, 1716–19

| Vessel | Origin | African purchase zone | Captain | Year | Debarked |
|---|---|---|---|---|---|
| Windsor | London | Loango (Congo) | Townshend | 1716 | 164 |
| Hope | London | Cabinda (Congo) | Cronker | 1716 | 188 |
| Arabella | London | Gambia | Bewes | 1717 | 188 |
| George | London | Loango | Malthus | 1717 | 245 |
| Saint Quintin | London | Loango | Hunt | 1717 | 294 |
| Sarah Galley | London | Madagascar | Bloome | 1717 | 347 |
| Opie Galley | ? | ? | ? | 1717 | 188 |
| Crown | London | Angola/Congo | Lone | 1718 | ? |
| Crown Galley | London | Angola/Congo | Hall | 1718 | 285 |
| Europe | London | Whydah | Dufay | 1718 | 312 |
| Thos. and Deb. | London | Whydah | Spencer | 1718 | 285 |
| Subtile | La Rochelle | Accra, Ghana | Geslin | 1718 | 111 |
| Kingston | London | Madagascar | Hamilton | 1719 | 208 |

Source: Trans-Atlantic Slave Trade Database.

returned to Plymouth on October 27, 1718, with far less Potosí silver than hoped, although, as Helen Paul has argued, the South Sea Company's slave trading was profitable and thus not a proximate cause of Britain's namesake bubble and stock market crash of 1720.[17]

Slave-ship quarantine or no, smallpox was not what was killing Buenos Aires residents in 1717, and the city's governor got medical experts to agree that people were dying from inadequate shelter and general poverty, not "plague or poisoned air." In the name of business, he withheld inconvenient facts that might spark panic along trade routes connecting Buenos Aires to the interior. The city council ordered cowhides sold for poor relief, and Jesuit fathers attended the sick, "as often Spaniards as Indians or Blacks." They went "out daily through the streets and plazas and on horseback toward the outskirts

17. Paul, South Sea Bubble.

of town, confessing the dying and relieving the rest as much as possible." An oxcart trucked victims' clothing and bedding outside town to be torched.[18]

Yet the putrid fevers lingered. On November 13, 1717, Buenos Aires's town council conceded that the "present epidemic is in full vigor," adding another 200 pesos from hide sales for sick relief. By January 1718 council members lamented a shortage of cowboys for the annual roundup. Soldiers at the city's fort were also felled. By August fraternity members shouldered the Virgin of the Rosary for a circumambulation in hopes of "lifting the painful lash that has stricken this miserable city." Another public supplication featured the city's patron, Saint Martin, and another, the Holy Trinity. By September Buenos Aires's aldermen bemoaned still more deaths, especially of Indigenous, Black, and Mulatto ranch hands. By some accounts the pandemic lingered for an excruciating sixteen months. It became difficult to distinguish death by peste from simple starvation. The "painful lash" finally lifted in December 1718.[19]

An episcopal visit to towns northwest of Buenos Aires found some stricken and others nearly untouched. The pathogen played leapfrog, a repeated pattern. Such was the case in and around the market towns of Santa Fe and Corrientes, despite steady interactions with Buenos Aires. Here and there a village or farm would be afflicted, or maybe a few urban households, but not whole cities. Similarly, the Jesuit missions of greater Paraguay were mostly spared. It is unclear why, but the fathers may have successfully quarantined infection at the outlying missions of Yapeyú and Santo Tomé on the middle Uruguay River.[20]

Meanwhile, the sickness spread to the inland trading hub of Córdoba, in central Argentina, where in 1718 and 1719 slaves on mule-breeding estancias fell by the hundreds—this according to their Jesuit owners. As demographic historian Aníbal Arcondo has shown, Indigenous ranch hands and housekeepers were also stricken. The Bavarian Jesuit José Klausner moved enslaved Africans north in 1718. He recalled in 1719, "Last year the plague raged terribly for three hundred leagues around [Córdoba], having been introduced by the English who embarked in Africa 600 Moors [sic] to resell them at

18. Biedma, *Acuerdos del extinguido cabildo*, 241–42, 254–57.
19. Ibid., 426, 474–75, 479, 524, 533–34, 587, 600, 614–16.
20. Livi-Bacci and Maeder, "Missions of Paraguay."

profit in America. Those poor people practically all got sick, and some died due to the long and cramped voyage. Only counting our college in the city [of Córdoba] and its haciendas, we lost 325 of those Black slaves, such that the countryside and ranches are deserted for lack of plantings."[21] Several Jesuits also died from the Gran Peste of 1718, as did lay brothers. Letters and wills from Córdoba's female convents likewise lament the ravages of the disease. Jesuit sources praise one of their own, Father Zsigmond Asperger, a Hungarian physician, with administering useful medicines, but we lack details on symptoms as well as therapies. No doubt influenced by the city's Jesuits, a novena was called by the Córdoba town council in honor of Saint Francis Xavier. Others were held for Saint Roch (patron of plague sufferers) and the martyrs Tiburtius, Valerian, and Maximus plus the Andes's own Virgin of Copacabana. Bullfights and cane jousts were halted on the September 30 feast of Saint Jerome, the city's patron, but not religious processions.

Next to be struck by the Gran Peste were northern towns dotting Tucumán Province, strung along the Camino Real, or "Royal Road," to Potosí, including Santiago del Estero and Salta, with Jujuy apparently spared, although not for long. Also hit was the highland town of Tarija, whose vineyards supplied Potosí with wine and brandy (a scourge bemoaned by Arzáns). In a 1725 census of the vineyards of Pilaya and Paspaya, Ann Zulawski found a steep population drop plus high incidence of Indigenous widows, single mothers, and orphans.[22]

Potosí, by far the largest and most commercially vibrant city in the region, was next in line, but also hit were the modest cities of La Plata and Oruro. The silver production in Oruro, which had nearly caught up to Potosí's by 1719, collapsed, dropping some 60 percent by 1721 due to a shortage of workers.[23] Preplague production levels were not restored until the 1750s. Jesuit writers tracked the pandemic to the Chiquitos Missions, east of Santa Cruz de la Sierra in

21. Arcondo, "Mortalidad general," esp. 71–75. Klausner backed his claims by enumerating drops in enslaved populations at two ranches plus the Jesuits' urban college of Monserrat: Santa Catalina (336 in 1718, then 252 in 1720, then 244 in 1721); La Candelaria (87 in 1718, then 76 in 1723); and the College of Monserrat (132 in 1718, then 90 in 1719). Death rates of 25–30 percent seem to have been typical (ibid.).
22. Zulawski, *They Eat from Their Labor*, 187–91.
23. Ibid., 109, 210. TePaske gives similar figures in *New World*, 192.

Bolivia's lowlands, and the peste seems then to have gone north to
La Paz and also west to the Pacific port of Arica, blasting through
nearby Arequipa and its hinterland before reaching Lima's outskirts,
where it depopulated the neighboring Sierra. Writing from the
mercury-mining town of Huancavelica on August 30, 1724, Jesuit
Manuel Toledo y Leiva noted, "the houses are mere monuments . . .
farms ruined, pueblos deserted." He estimated greater Peru's Indigenous death toll at more than 150,000.[24]

Lima seems to have been spared, and the pandemic does not
appear to have reached Quito, much less Bogotá, the north Andes'
main population centers. Far less fortunate was the old Inca capital
of Cuzco, long connected to Potosí via the coca trade. According to
witnesses, Cuzco was devastated, hit at least as hard as Potosí, if
not harder. A detailed description of the peste in Cuzco is offered in
translation here.[25] Franciscan missions in Peru's eastern lowlands
were afflicted too, but these were isolated populations already suffering numerous maladies.[26]

For the story of Cuzco, we rely on Creole chronicler and priest
Diego de Esquivel y Navia (ca. 1700–1779). Although their styles dif-
fer, Esquivel's *Chronological News of the Great City of Cuzco* bears
comparison with Arzáns's *History of the Imperial Villa of Potosí*.
Esquivel adopts an enlightened tone, sticking to the "facts," although
as a priest he could not resist sermonizing. If we may trust Esquivel,
the bishopric of Cuzco was crushed, with some twenty thousand city
dwellers succumbing to the Gran Peste and as many as forty thousand more dying in the countryside. As in greater Potosí, the vast
majority of victims were native Andeans.

More recognizably scientific responses to the pandemic came from
Lima, capital of the viceroyalty and home to several world-class physicians and highly learned figures. Among them was Sicilian medical
doctor Federico Bottoni, who included a description of the pestilence

24. Toledo y Leiva, quoted in Vargas Ugarte, *Pareceres jurídicos*, 168–83, esp. 179.
25. A brief account is given in Colin, *Cuzco*, 32–38, and I use Colin's transcription
of a document in the Archivo General de Indias (hereafter AGI) for chapter 5, "The
Cure." Special thanks to Prof. Gabriela Ramos for kindly pointing me to this source
when I was unable to visit the archives because of COVID-19 travel restrictions.
26. See Santos Guerrero, "Epidemias y sublevaciones." See also Cameron Jones, *In
Service of Two Masters*, 31.

in his treatise on the human circulatory system, published in 1723 and translated here. It offers a rare description of symptoms.

Accounts of the Gran Peste's descent on the city of Arequipa suggest it was nearly as hard-hit as Potosí and Cuzco. The "contagion" did not discriminate, emptying Indigenous towns for miles around and leaving dozens of wealthy townsfolk's urban mansions entirely abandoned, doors and shutters banging in the pestilential wind.

As is clear from this overview, South America's Great Pandemic of 1717–22 depopulated town and country as it leapfrogged from the Atlantic port of Buenos Aires through the Andean highlands to the Pacific coast, killing something on the order of two hundred thousand people or more. A December 29, 1720, report from Lima to the king already claimed a death toll of four hundred thousand for Peru's "twenty-five provinces."[27] Greater Peru's highland core was hardest hit, losing roughly half its urban and rural Indigenous populations.

Trade between Upper Peru's silver producers and the slavers, contraband traders, yerba maté growers, and mule breeders of the Río de la Plata was disrupted for many years, as Arzáns claimed near the end of his life. The region's economic motor, the Imperial Villa of Potosí, was left sputtering, and a new wave of disease blasted through the Paraguayan missions and much of the Río de la Plata in the early 1730s.

As Michèle Colin, Ann Wightman, and Ward Stavig show, for the vast bishopric of Cuzco, the plague-induced population crash of 1720 had lasting consequences. It was devastating for native Andeans in the short term, but it also enabled Crown officials to alter counting

---

27. Colin, *Cuzco*, 37n32. This anonymous report reads,

> The universal calamity that the twenty-five provinces of this kingdom have suffered with the destruction caused by a terrible plague has been among the greatest experienced since its discovery, as it has burned through towns, villas, and cities to the point of leaving them ravaged and barren of their original inhabitants, such that, according to the reports from priests and governors, the number of dead has risen to four hundred thousand, there remaining in many places nothing but bare walls to enumerate, such is the severity with which God has punished our sins, and this excessive tribulation continues in Cuzco, seeing in its streets every day a bloody theater of cadavers torn apart by dogs for lack of anyone among the living willing to give them burial, possessed by the horror in which they hold the violence of the contagion. In this city [of Lima] there is expected no less lamentable a tragedy should divine mercy not spare us. (My translation.)

mechanisms controlling tribute and mita obligations.[28] Backing up, Stavig found mention of 1719 pandemic deaths of Cuzco-area mita workers in the Potosí parishes of Concepción and San Sebastián: twelve individuals from Pomacanchis, twenty-three from Coporaque, and thirteen from Pueblo Nuevo, far above prepandemic death rates in their home pueblos, all south of Cuzco. Stavig also found victims' names: "Families were decimated or wiped out: for instance, Pablo Luntu and his wife, Nicolasa Casa; Francisco Cayagua, age thirteen, followed shortly after by his father and mother; and María Colquema and her son, Melchor."[29]

The cacique don Juan Bautista Uri-Siri of Carangas petitioned the regional court on behalf of all of Potosí's mita captains "that the mita be suspended until the plague ceases in Potosí." The pandemic accompanied returning migrant workers north, as Stavig continues:

> In 1719–1720 the pandemic that swept the Andes worked to its deadly conclusion in rural Cuzco. Between 1682 and 1702 deaths in Ccatcca, a community near the Paucartambo-Quispicanchis border, averaged between 20 and 25 per year. In 1720, between June and August, 469 people died. After this nobody recorded the mortalities, because the priest and those in charge of the major [religious confraternities] had died. . . . The community of Quiquijana suffered similar devastation. The epidemic raged for nearly half a year, after which it was reported that "there are very few people in the pueblo, for which cause all the plantings of maize and wheat, potatoes, and other vegetables have been lost, not having people to harvest them. They have also lost the royal tributes because of the death of the Indians and . . . caciques."[30]

28. Ibid.; Wightman, *Indigenous Migration*, 42–43, chap. 7; Stavig, *World of Túpac Amaru*. The peste killed so many that tributes were suspended and the *retasa*, or "recount," in the late 1720s shifted the whole tax structure to reflect reality, the first major change since Toledo set the system up to distinguish *originarios* (locals) from *forasteros* (outsiders). Now the lack of distinction rendered more men eligible for mita service, a major change. Huancavelica's mining mita pool shrank, but Potosí's expanded, altering migration incentives.
29. Stavig, *World of Túpac Amaru*, 193.
30. Ibid., 193, 227. Stavig cites Burga, "La crisis del XVIII," and his own 1988 *Hispanic American Historical Review* article for this. The archival source provided in his notes is Cuzco's departmental archive, "1720 peste."

Ordinary people were not listed, but titled headmen were named
for Spanish records:

> Don Francisco Niño, don Martín Tiraquimbo, don Melchor
> Guamansauni, don Tomás Ramos, and don Alonso Orcoguarana
> who were [paramount chiefs] and governors of this pueblo
> are dead, they died in the *peste* . . . and of the same fate have
> died all the [subchiefs] and [regional bosses] like Francisco de
> Estrada who died without one member of his family remaining,
> and in the same manner Mateo Pichu with all his family, don
> Gabriel Cusigualpa, Agustín de Rado, don Eugenio Ninamalco
> and others, and don Blas Chinche who was [chief magistrate]
> with the said don Melchor Guamansauni, and those that were
> placed [in office] afterwards by your mercy, Señor Corregidor
> [Lord Governor], they also died, as did all the [aldermen and
> justices], and the only [district bosses] that remain alive are don
> Miguel Quera and don Fernando Vitorino.[31]

Stavig notes how survivors sold land to raise money for tribute as
royal officials took more.

Adrian Pearce expanded on these Cuzco-area findings to show
how the Gran Peste had profound macroregional implications. It
sparked the first major Andean census in many decades, providing
historians with a clearer picture of demographic trends.[32] Yet, as
Pearce also explains, for native Andeans the drawn-out 1724–40
census was not benign, and, rather like the Slave Trade Database, its
raw numbers both quantify and mask a dark regime of racialized
exploitation.

Curiously, the old archbishop-viceroy, Fray Diego Morcillo, played
a bridge role. When the prince of Santo Buono left Lima in 1719,
Morcillo was again named interim viceroy of Peru, as Arzáns notes.
Having been feted by Potosí industrialists, Morcillo resisted a new
"permanent" census that might harm powerful interests, even as
he allowed anguished Indigenous headmen to submit temporary
recounts to alleviate postplague tribute and labor demands. Under
layers of legalese one gains a sense of this desperation in a petition

31. Stavig, *World of Túpac Amaru*, 230.
32. Pearce, "Peruvian Population Census."

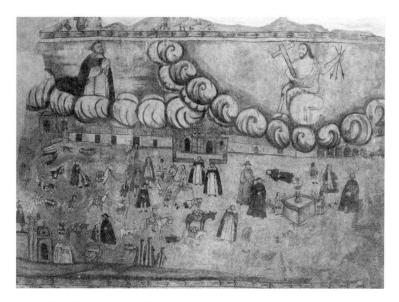

FIG. 4. Detail from the *Pandemic Mural* at Ccatcca, Peru. Courtesy of Raúl Montero Quispe.

filed in Lima on July 13, 1722, by two caciques from Carangas, near the present-day border between Bolivia and Chile:

> Don Melchor de la Cruz Sacama and don Pedro Sacama, governors and caciques of the pueblo of San Pedro de Totora, province of Carangas, for themselves and in name of the other paramount chiefs and other native people of the town, and as proof of their presentation and relation before the viceroy that, his lordship having ordered the royal officials of this kingdom to see that the corregidors of each province draw up [new] lists of the Indians who survive after having suffered from the general epidemic, the same that has been observed and practiced thus, but not in the said province of Carangas due to carelessness and omission by those who should have carried them out, from which have resulted and shall result in future notable injustices, it being impossible for [we caciques] to comply with the tribute submissions based on the old head counts, due to the lack of Indians caused by the aforementioned epidemic. And they ask and plead that it would be right to order the corregidor

[of Carangas] to undertake a recount of the said Indians, original inhabitants and transients, who happen to remain after the passing of the contagion that has brought such ruin upon them.[33]

Thus, it was only with the 1724 arrival of yet another viceroy, the Marquis of Castelfuerte, that new, official Indigenous head counts were registered, harbingers of more regimented and inflexible reforms to come. As Pearce amply shows, "Viceroy Hardcastle" personified a new era in which local elites would not easily purchase royal favors and in which the extraction of Potosí silver paid for with Indigenous blood and sweat grew more systematic. The great Andean pandemic gave way to "disaster imperialism," an outcome familiar to sufferers of another great outbreak on the other side of the Atlantic.

## A French Connection?

Observers in Potosí, Cuzco, and other parts of South America called "their" pandemic a peste, or "plague," sometimes referring back (as did Arzáns) to the Great Plague of the 1340s. History seemed to be repeating itself worldwide, as plague (*Yersinia pestis*) hit Marseille, France, just as so-called peste blew through the Andes. Whatever their specific causes, the results of these plagues were similar. Between 1720 and 1722 Marseille lost some fifty thousand people, or nearly half its population.

It all began in May 1720, when the ship *Grand Saint-Antoine* docked in Marseille's Vieux Port after a trading voyage to Syria and Palestine by way of Cyprus. During a stop in Livorno, on the Tuscan coast, an inventory of dead crew members signaled contagion aboard,

33. Sánchez-Albornoz, *Indios y tributos*, 170n9, cites Archivo General de la Nación, Lima, sec. 9, doc.10.9.1 (my translation). In his demographic history of Tapacarí's pueblos (Quillacollo, Tiquipaya, Sipesipe, Calliri) near Cochabamba, Sánchez-Albornoz noted a near 25 percent drop in male tributaries between 1683 (2,211) and 1732 (1,583), by which time rebound occurred (164). Sánchez-Albornoz added that the 1719 peste hit *forasteros* harder than *originarios*, but the former were incorporated into communities, as Pearce shows and the petition suggests (166). It was a counting issue. The upshot: Indigenous populations dropped steadily from at least 1573 to just after 1719 before a long, slow recovery (170). Thanks to Sinclair Thomson for this source.

but upon reaching Marseille the ship was not quarantined according to law. Prominent city merchants with a stake in the cargo sought to unload their goods duty-free. Improperly handled, the *Grand Saint-Antoine* disgorged an army of rats and fleas into the unsuspecting city.

Plague was believed to originate in "the Orient," specifically the Levant but also in the Maghreb. Despite this belief, seconded by historians of medicine, merchants hated waiting forty days to realize profits from fabrics, spices, drugs, and other exotic merchandise. The temptation to skip quarantine was irresistible. Rumors of a death ship were countered by official claims in July 1720 of "containment" or that the illness killing the *Saint-Antoine*'s crew was not plague.

But it *was* plague, and it was not contained. The bacillus ravaged Marseille, soon infecting neighboring towns and prompting royal intervention in the form of draconian travel restrictions, troop mobilization, health checkpoints, *cordons sanitaires* (including stone walls), and quarantine orders, all overseen by a new health council in Paris. Plague doctors donned elaborate masks and gowns, a kind of waxed-linen hazmat suit. The airborne poison was said to be "sticky."

News from Marseille traveled quickly (for the time), and beginning in August 1720 King Philip V of Spain and his ministers issued "global" warnings and pleas to pray for the monarch's French cousins. A copycat health council convened in Madrid, and, as Cindy Ermus has shown, the threat of plague from Marseille enabled Philip V's ministers to test-drive enlightened absolutism in the port city of Cádiz, gateway to the Indies.[34] Unaware of the Andean pandemic, the king dispatched decrees warning of infected French ships.

Things should not have gotten this far. Marseille, like other Mediterranean cities, had a quarantine hospital and a health bureau in contact with port authorities in Venice, Genoa, Livorno, and Barcelona.[35] Control of these institutions in Marseille, as Junko Takeda shows, was contested under Louis XV, and passion bred blindness. Skipped quarantine plus port authorities' downplaying of the plague

34. See Ermus, "Plague of Provence"; Ermus, "Spanish Plague"; and Varela Peris, "Junta Suprema de Sanidad." See also Archivo de la Real Chancillería de Valladolid, Spain, Cédulas y Pragmáticas, c. 22:35. The king ordered public supplications to the Virgin Mary, Saint Michael, Saint Sebastian, and Saint Roch.

35. Cipolla, *Fighting the Plague*.

in its first days seemed to be the "true" causes of the devastating outbreak.[36]

Blame aside, Marseille's public health officials, backed by the king, issued decrees as the epidemic spiraled out of control. Physicians and surgeons who fled to the provinces were ordered to return to practice or lose their licenses. Farmers were forbidden from diverting water from the city's main supply lines for irrigation, as it was needed for public fountains and sewerage. Bakers could not bake white bread and biscuits from relief supplies of grain and flour. And perhaps most bizarrely, butchers were not to inflate sheep and cattle carcasses with their mouths, an alleged means of spreading plague.[37]

Dealing with the sick, the dying, and the dead became a logistical nightmare, and volunteers were few. A shortage of horses, carts, and harnesses added to the confusion, and rural folk refused to come to Marseille to move bodies—at any price. Desperate city officials pleaded, "We need 'crows' [i.e., doctors or morticians donning beak-like masks] to remove corpses from houses, and yet whatever excessive payment we offer, the most miserable flee such a perilous job and go to great lengths to avoid doing it. We need peasants to dig graves, and yet none want to work at it because they are overtaken by fear and horror. The aldermen are forced to bend over backward to effectively convince some and to use force and rigor with others."[38]

Galley slaves manned front lines as tensions rose regarding religious processions and public devotion. The people spoke with their feet, trusting God and the saints:

> [Regarding] August 16, Saint Roch's feast day, which has always been solemnized in Marseille in order to preserve it from the plague, the [mayor] Marquis of Pilles and the aldermen, in order to avoid the spread [of the disease], wished to prohibit the procession that takes place every year, during which the bust and relics of this saint are carried about. But they must give in to the people's outcry, as they are furious with devotion when they fear a scourge as terrible as the plague, of which they already see the horrible impact. The

36. Takeda, Between Crown and Commerce, 131–57.
37. Jauffret, Pièces historiques, 51–52.
38. Ibid., 55–56.

> [marquis and aldermen] even think it proper to participate
> in the procession [themselves] with all their halberdiers and
> guards, so as to prevent anyone from following them or form-
> ing a crowd and creating confusion.[39]

Here was a way to participate in pious display while also enforc-
ing social distancing. The Crown, meanwhile, enacted massive grain
purchases, hospital and temporary infirmary construction, production
and warehousing of medical supplies, and detailed data collection.
Unfortunately, containment efforts came too late. Although the
plague did not ravage all of France thanks in part to physical barriers,
the disease rolled on into 1722, killing many in Aix and other parts of
Provence and even Languedoc.

Observers of the 1720 Marseille plague likened it to earlier outbreaks, placing it in historical context before the last corpse was cold.
As will be seen, Potosí chronicler Bartolomé Arzáns did likewise,
interspersing descriptions of the disease ravaging his hometown
in 1719 with narratives of the Black Plague of the 1340s. By inter-
calating symptoms and effects of the two ailments, Arzáns reveals
uncanny similarities while also highlighting differences. Was the
Gran Peste of the Andes even plague?

The bubonic plague was spread by fleas drawing the *Yersinia*
bacillus from infected rats, and exposure led to a quick and ugly death
marked by fever, black bumps, swollen lymph nodes, secretions, and
bruise-like rashes. Mortality rates averaged 10 to 30 percent in a
given outbreak, but they could go higher among malnourished or
otherwise compromised populations. The great "plague" of Potosí
(and greater Spanish South America) was not much prettier in terms
of symptoms, and its mortality was similar, especially among the
poor.

Enlightened physicians lent a hand, but both new and old inter-
pretations of plague circa 1720 were based on humoral theory. The
new "rational" view was optimistic, at the Panglossian extreme argu-
ing that plague was simply a physical manifestation of panic. Others
spoke of a "foreign yeast" that flourished in bad air. Indeed, many
blamed plagues and other pandemics on "venomous air," or miasma,
a view shared by ancient Greeks. Some victims were more susceptible

---

39. Ibid., 56.

to the "venom" (or "yeast") in this bad air due to their own bodily disequilibrium, which might be remedied with bloodletting, emetics, sweats, and plasters. Some of these therapies were benign, but they could also be deadly. As for pharmaceuticals, King Louis XV personally promoted one plague prescription, published in September 1720. The "patent," which the king had purchased, was freely distributed in the interest of public health.[40] We do not know if it saved lives, but the "open-access" recipe was an Alkermes, or *aurifique minéral*, a class of cure-alls containing heavy metals. The king's cure amounted to a distilled blend of gunpowder and "Hungarian antimony," administered in small doses dissolved in wine and sweetened with sugar. The medicine was said to cleanse the blood and intestines of "impurities," also "quickening the urine." Fortunately, it was not easy to make.[41]

But all this was superficial. Pandemic periodicity, according to prevailing theory, had deeper causes, lining up with historical (and thus cosmic) rhythms. Miasma alone was not to blame for the plague or pandemic—or, rather, miasmas arose only in specific moments or conjunctures. For many, echoing Thucydides, plague coincided with political disequilibrium and moral corruption. A pandemic or plague outbreak was a kind of corrective mass purge. Over time medical astrologers added celestial factors to the mix, a theme picked up by Arzáns in Potosí.[42]

Moral decay bred scapegoats too, and in France, Italy, and else-where in the Catholic world, women were targeted, as were foreigners, Jews, Gypsies, and other minorities. As will be seen in the case of Potosí and as was also claimed in 1720 Marseille, women of allegedly loose morals and tight-fitting dress were magnets of divine retribution. If plague was caused by social, political, and moral disorder, so also its results, at least in the short term. Pandemics disrupted natural hierarchies, dissolved friendships, and eroded filial piety. At its worse, peste "deranged" both the individual body and the body politic.[43]

40. Hammond and Sturgill, "French Plague Recipe."
41. Ibid., 594–95.
42. See Suárez, *Astros, humores, y cometas.*
43. Eamon, "Cannibalism and Contagion" (special thanks to Farren Yero for this reference). See also Colin Jones, "Plague and Its Metaphors"; and Slack, "Responses to Plague."

What were the consequences of the great 1720–22 Marseille plague? As Takeda shows, Marseille, aside from bearing the brunt of one of Europe's last Great Plague disasters, was already wracked by social and political division, pitting those who argued for the benefits of cosmopolitanism and global commerce against those who saw foreign trade as a corrupting factor, one that encouraged not only avarice and waste but also "Turkish" vices and "foreign" ailments. Amid recovery, Marseille's cosmopolitan identity was shelved and its old "noncommercial republican" identity revived. Civic virtue demanded elite self-sacrifice, moral rectitude, and profligate religious piety. Amid fear and social atomization, this response could be cast as a restoration, reaffirming the near at hand, if not rejecting the foreign, and loudly reinforcing a shared sense of communal self-reliance and pious Roman Catholicism. Yet Takeda found that Crown officials exploited Marseille's misfortunes to cement absolutist power just the same, even as the king's bitter medicine failed.[44]

Something similar was brewing in the Andes, just as global disease concerns converged. In April 1722 officials in the equatorial city of Quito received a decree prohibiting commerce with French vessels on the Pacific coast. Another decree arrived in December, specifically banning merchandise from Marseille.[45] This was all rather late, but Spain's colonial officials touted their importance as protectors of "public health," a term that, as in France, was current.

News of the Marseille plague crept around the globe much like disease itself. On June 20, 1723, having finally received the royal proclamations from December 1720 and August 1721, officials in Manila, the capital of the Spanish Philippines, banned French ships. Philip V's decrees would be enforced "to protect the health of the Natives."[46] Coincidentally, back in Spain, a royal edict reopened commerce with France just a few weeks later, on July 12, 1723, "the plague having ceased in Marseille."[47]

44. Takeda, *Between Crown and Commerce*, 180–96.
45. AGI, Quito, leg. 129, no. 23, fol. 85. The repeal of the ban on commerce with France is in AGI, Quito, leg. 23, no. 9.
46. AGI, Filipinas, leg. 139, no. 20, fol. 1 (cover page).
47. Archivo de la Real Chancillería de Valladolid, Spain, Cédulas y Pragmáticas, c. 23, no. 9.

## The Story

Three years ago heaven sent a warning, horrendous fire, presaging calamity. The comet—maverick sun, crazy sun—pointed its tail at the mountain of Potosí.[48]

Thus begins Eduardo Galeano's brief summary of the 1719 pandemic, in *Faces and Masks*, volume 2 of *Memory of Fire*, digesting the account of Bartolomé Arzáns. By contrast, the present book administers a full dose of Arzáns's reflections on Potosí's "Gran Peste." Although he suggests the disease originated in Europe (without naming Marseille), Arzáns connects it to the slave trade via Buenos Aires. He opens with a series of omens, predictions, and portents before describing the sickness, which sounds like a hemorrhagic fever. Detailing symptoms, he cites a physician who, as far as we know, did not exist.[49]

Arzáns then describes a veritable blitz of religious processions, including some to "plague protector" Saint Roch, a reminder that, despite awareness of contagion ("just by looking at a sick person you could get it," Arzáns warns), there seems to have been little interest in social distancing. And whereas Marseille's plague doctors wore maximum personal protective equipment, Potosí's priests strode boldly unto the breach, as if to test their sanctity. Clerics were expected to care for the sick, inspired by plague fighters like Roch and the recently canonized Saint John of God. Interspersed with processions and other pious acts are moral asides or cases, peculiar or uncanny events that feature either sinful or pious individuals and the horrifying or miraculous consequences of their actions. The narrative hovers over personal responsibility.

In describing those who cared for the sick or otherwise provided relief, Arzáns goes out of his way to praise pious men and a few women (one a champion breast feeder), most of them members of Potosí's Hispanic elite. For the author, these individuals' charitable deeds were worthy of memorializing in writing, whereas the majority of Indigenous victims, the city's poorest and most vulnerable, remain all but nameless, pitiful exempla. Either way, Arzáns makes clear that the poor and Indigenous suffered most, by a huge margin.

48. Galeano, *Faces and Masks*, 18.
49. Arzáns often cites imaginary authorities on technical matters, as if to add credibility.

There are other parallels with more recent pandemics, but mostly Arzáns's early eighteenth-century account evokes a radically different world in which comets foretold calamities, "indecent" female dress outraged "divine justice," and the repeated parading of statues of the Virgin Mary, Jesus Christ, and dozens of saints in tightly packed crowds of believers was assumed effective. Processions to Saint Rose of Lima may have been linked to female chastity, and those to the Virgin of Copacabana, a local saint, may have been aimed at Indigenous protection. Relics or holy remains of Saint Sebastian were paraded to spread his alleged healing powers, but, as will be seen, every saint in town got a workout.

Despite constant supplications, the pandemic raged on for nearly a full year in Potosí, and the bodies piled up such that new cemeteries and ossuaries had to be built in and around town. When it was all over, at least a third of Potosí's and of greater Peru's already beaten-down population, primarily its Indigenous majority, lay dead. Throughout the ordeal Arzáns asks what price the world's most famous mining boomtown must pay for its accumulated, perhaps incalculable sins. His answer? God only knows.

# 1

## Pandemic in Potosí

### Chapter XLVI

For the sins of this Imperial Villa, God destroyed it with an epidemic pestilence. Also included are some notable incidents that were seen in this destructive episode and other things that occurred in this year.[1]

Humans do not wish to stop persuading themselves that the pains of the soul are many times the origin of exterior illnesses such that the body cannot enjoy health when the soul is suffering the fevers of vice. I have said as much many times in the course of this *History*, always fearing and always predicting for this Imperial Villa some ruin or punishment for its sins, and if for not having come to light already they might be excused, but forgiveness is not possible when accused by one's own conscience, the preachers and missionaries having exhorted and warned them repeatedly of the wrath of God, [threatening] losses in their business enterprises, portentous events, the present poverty, and they foresaw many other ills. For this, then, all of us inhabitants [of Potosí] were punished with a terrible illness, as I will describe with all possible brevity, since if I were to write about this great calamity in all its circumstances, and in particular about the exemplary portents, it would be necessary to fill another of the large volumes that make up this *History*. . . .

He who does not repress evil and punish misdeeds when he can, enables them, and it is also true that by not prohibiting crime when

---

1. Chapter XLVI from Arzáns de Orsúa y Vela, *Historia*, 3:77–103 (pt. 1, bk. 10, chaps. 46–49). This and all translations from the Spanish are by Kris Lane.

one can, one asks for it. In not rushing to evacuate ill humors from the human body, one brings about corruption and death (and the present year matches this experience). Thus the body of the republic will come to perish if those who govern are not quickly removed should they fail to administer the necessary medicines in their sentences. Human justice punishes public and scandalous sins, because, if not, divine justice will do so with such generality that not even the innocents shall be spared when the guilty irritate the divine. So says the current experience.

Sunday, January 8 of this year, this villa celebrated the reception into the fold of our holy mother Roman Catholic Church one Cristóbal Baltasar Gorote, a German by nation, from one of the cantons, native of Hanover, who, by way of a parcel of enslaved Africans, arrived from Buenos Aires with the English monopolists. After having been presented to the illustrious and most excellent lord archbishop [Morcillo] of La Plata, and his eminence having given order for what ought to be done in this instance, there was brought together a tribunal of the Holy Inquisition, whose commissioner [stood witness as the German] publicly abjured heresies and proclaimed the articles of the faith that up to that time he had denied. His godfather was don Martín de Echevarría, knight of Santiago, and the ceremony was attended by the town council, prelates, and all the nobles and common people, a function carried out with great solemnity and enjoyment, seeing the desire with which he requested and received our holy faith. His conversion was spurred by having seen the mortification practiced by the Carmelite nuns in the Potosí convent, having entered to visit a sick woman, and this left him stunned, seeing and pondering how among young, beautiful, and delicate women without sins there was such mortification, and he asked outside what that meant, or what guilt they carried so as to treat themselves this way, and he was satisfied inasmuch as was possible (not knowing our language), given to understand that they did it of their own will to gain heaven, to which he later responded, "If these ladies do only this in order to gain heaven, then those of us who go about only in search of silver without doing similar things will undoubtedly be condemned." Thus opening the door, with this [reflection] his conversion was facilitated and he requested baptism, and after [he was] well instructed, it was granted him *sub conditione* with great solemnity and concourse [of people], as it was such a novelty in this villa.

In town at the start of this year were don José de la Quintana, don Miguel de Zubiegui, and other Basques and [residents of] some other nations [i.e., regions] of Spain who had just arrived, and they were so caught up in the sale of their merchandise in order to get back to Spain that they were overcome as always with that terrible Spanish greed, worse than that of other foreign nations, such that what a Frenchman would sell for ten pesos the Spaniard is not content with thirty. Thus they collected millions in silver coins, bars, and worked items, finally leaving the local inhabitants without any means of remediating the most grave necessity that was coming on with all speed in the form of a mortal plague. These men showed themselves to have forgotten common sense: so impassive were they that they did not realize what their fierce greed would do to the poor, the widow, and the orphan. An avaricious heart is never satisfied, and, just as fortune might give one all the possessions in the universe, it still pains one to see what others possess, and it saddens one to not have everything for oneself. It was not unjust to sell goods and collect silver, but not with such extreme avarice. So now divine justice prepared its punishment for the sinners of this villa and sent in advance these harvesters of the fruit of its mountain so as to catch them without that means of relief.

The rains this year were also severe and noxious to this villa, which was taken as an omen of the coming calamity, as the downpours began on December 21 of the preceding year [1718] and continued with great fury to the beginning of autumn (which in our hemisphere is March 20), destroying many houses and killing many, the rising rivers doing considerable damage. The church and monastery of Saint Dominic were about to collapse entirely, and thus they begged mercy of the Virgin of the Rosary with a very devout procession, and God was served to mitigate this punishment—only to release an even greater one soon after.

In addition to this omen (fourth time this year) there preached on Holy Thursday in the monastery of Saint Augustine one evening the reverend father missionary Fray Francisco Romero regarding the life of Saint Mary of Egypt with its eloquent but also startling doctrine, warning the sinners of this villa with threats of divine justice for their repeated sins, but it was all fruitless, as the presumptuous sinner hopes in vain, because without facing down difficulties one abuses mercy and brings on divine justice against oneself.² Such clear calls for repentance served for nothing, and thus it was quite sad the state into which the villa was putting itself with its public sins of sensuality, greed, larceny, homicide, injustice, and more, facing threats of worse ills by not quickly seeking remedy. This was made extremely difficult due to the little or no fear with which the evildoers did their evil, seeing also that their misdeeds were helped along by those who could have prevented them, and the presumption with which they practiced them made their "illness" most desperate and almost incurable.

These warnings came not only from the mouth of this apostolic missionary but also from that of the very reverend father Fray Juan de Águilar of the Order of Preachers (son of this villa, having received in this very year from Rome the title of apostolic preacher). And he preached "mission" [i.e., to nonbelievers] at the start of this year in the smaller parish of Saint Francis (where he was interim priest during the trip to Rome of the most reverend father maestro Fray Bernardino Solórzano). [Águilar] predicted the evil that would fall on this villa if it did not repent its vices. His words were clear, full of truth and stripped of all affectation, directed to the honor of God and to the detestation of all sins. Seven years had now passed in which every Friday evening he performed the *vía sacra* [stations of the cross] in his church of preachers [Santo Domingo] and later preached with great spirit, exhorting repentance for sins, as he went on doing. This devotion of the *vía sacra* was introduced after the lamentable event that was the sacrilegious death of the very reverend father Fray Sancho Marañón, prior of his monastery, as is told in its place in this *History*, and always in his sermons he predicted a punishment. If this is what corresponded with [that crime], may God be praised, as so piously he punishes this and other grave sins.

In the same way the venerable Jesuit fathers in their Easter sermons and in their annual mission, which is done to honor Christ our Lord in the month of September, warned this villa in their sermons as a result of the scandalous sins its inhabitants committed. The virtue ascribed to these venerable men made them discreet in their

---

2. Saint Mary of Egypt was a repentant prostitute.

reprehensions. Without failing to reveal themselves zealous defenders of God's honor, they showed love in the confessional while also demonstrating abhorrence of vices, seasoning their admonishments with the salt of prudence, applying without excess the remedy for the illnesses of sin, and indeed the greatest skill of a preacher consists of identifying wounds and applying the proper medicine with tenderness and care, such that the resistance of the patient does not negate the art nor defile the doctrine.

Thus did these apostolic preachers execute their duty, but nothing bore fruit because the hearts they found were hardened by such a range of sins. Thus, what could one expect other than destruction and death? Oh damned villa! And how much evil awaits you, as you do not now value the worship and veneration that must always be shown to God our Lord and to his Most Holy Mother and to his saints; none of the charity that you so desire [will come your way], because you lack the essential, which is to love and fear God! I know well that you are my compass and cradle [speaking to Potosí, his hometown], and for this reason I would like to refrain from writing of the grave outcomes caused by your sins, but it is divine will that does not permit it, since I remain alive when so many compatriots and foreign visitors were so cruelly despoiled by death.

Sighs and abundant tears shall accompany my pen, and I will continue only so as to reach the end of my much-delayed *History* (although I have written of such lamentable destructions); not one of them [i.e., these earlier episodes] bore such consequences and produced so many trials, nor such a high number of inhabitants who perished nor subsequent damages experienced. Let us proceed, then, starting by continuing with the omens that were witnessed, the natural causes that came together, several more public contemptuous acts against God, and scandalous dishonesties that finally provoked divine justice.

In chapter 42 of this tenth book [of the *History of Potosí*], we noted how on Sunday, according to the calendar, June 14 of that year 1716, at half past nine at night, there passed over this villa a great light, exhalation, or whatever it was, which no one could quite distinguish, whose form (as I said there) was elongated, exhibiting a bit more width at the head, the tail petering out, and the brightness it showed was equal to that of the sun, of a color whiter than citrine, although speckled, the sound frightening like a clap of thunder, and going on its path from north to south, the same coming from the direction of La Plata [today Sucre], where it also passed alongside around nine at night.[3] I already mentioned in the cited passage other consequences of this matter, and how in passing over the Cerro Rico it caused it to tremble, and then it continued on its path toward the provinces of Tucumán and Buenos Aires, as we later learned.

The fear of all was great, and at the same time the shared ignorance of what it was and the various discourses that arose about it were such that, if mine alone and my pen had prevailed (although indeterminately), [it would have been agreed] that it was a sign from heaven with which men are typically warned to fear justice. What I can say now is that, after reading ancient and modern histories by many authors, poets, and orators, I have found that to this day never in the world were seen such phenomena in the air that were not followed (within one, two, or, at most, three years) by notable disasters and calamities in the areas where such planets or fires threatened, and thus the poets tend to call comets *dirus*, which means cruel and sanguinary, as Virgil called them; Lucan called them *sidas*, or "fearful star"; Pontanus [called them] "threateners"; Pliny, "scary ones"; Angelus Policianus, "sad ones."

If that frightening fire that passed over this villa was an omen presaging its destruction, at two years and eight months afterward, it came to pass at a time when only a few still feared it, and many made light of it, and some said it was ball lightning [*globo*], when it was far from being that. Very often God wills that such prodigies appear in the air, portents and signs (of which I could provide innumerable examples if I did not fear much delay) so as to awaken us from the carelessness with which we live and to warn us that we have angered him, [seeking] to revoke the sentence that he has issued against us, if with fruits worthy of penitence we would know how to reach him, just as those of Ninevah did.[4] They signify, then, these signs (or the malign quality of the impressions that the exhalations of the land by force of the same planets, which are, as the astrologers say, the comets' parents, tending to form in the supreme region of the air, their vapors catching fire there since they are close to the sphere of fire), they signify, as I am going to say: famines, plagues, droughts, deaths

3. Arzáns de Orsúa y Vela, *Historia*, 3:54.
4. Jonah 3 (King James Version).

of princes, the fall of kingdoms and republics, wars and internal rebellions, atrocious and imponderable events, and greater is the evil they signify when they come from a poorer quality or type of planet or planets by whose influence they are engendered.[5] There also occur other portents in the land, such as monstrous births in humans and animals, to the same effect, from women giving birth to some with two heads stuck together or stuck together at the chest or shoulders, others with four arms or legs, or others with notable deformities, among them many who lack some part of the body, and, although this comes from an overabundance or lack of semen, ordinarily this occurs as prognostication of various tribulations, of which one could produce infinite examples.[6] In this Imperial Villa of Potosí at the beginning of the month of January of this year, it happened, in the blocks of the San Pedro parish, that one Monday morning there passed through an alley a certain priest, who upon seeing an Indian in the doorstep of a hut, he was soon called on with great begging to baptize a newborn. He entered with great charity, that priest, when the wife of that Indian thrust into his arms a baby boy who had two heads (the one normal and the other emerging from the breastbone), each facing the other. The priest was astonished, and with the unexpected shock he did not see that the attached baby had two little hands minus the wrist joints, as the parents told him.[7] Faced with such an unseen novelty, this priest did not dare to apply water, not knowing if he was to perform [one or] two baptisms. In this instance he had not read the rules set up for such monsters, and thus, filled with astonishment, he told the parents he would return once he had determined what was to be done since there were two heads. With this he went off and returned at two in the afternoon, but he found the hut without the newborn, nor its parents, nor any other person great or small who could explain their absence, from which he came to believe that these ignorant folk, with the fear of this novelty and not wanting to show it to their parish priest, as it might have been seen as their crime, they all hid themselves,

5. As Aníbal Arcondo noted in "Mortalidad general," the Jesuit Dobrizhoffer spoke of comets in the Río de la Plata just after Arzáns. See also Dobrizhoffer, *Account of the Abipones*, 2:247; in Spanish: Dobrizhoffer, *Historia de los abipones*, 2:241.
6. On "monstrous births," see Pueyo, *Cuerpos plegables*.
7. A similar dilemma appears in Rivilla Bonet y Pueyo, *Desvíos de la naturaleza*.

knowing that this priest would go and tell others and thus perhaps the newborn would remain unbaptized, and, as some Indians are of the barbaric sort and they kill their own, this may have happened, as no more was found out about it.

Lasciviousness was so entrenched among the youth of this villa that none remembered that they had a God to fear nor a soul to look after, with which this vice, being so contrary to virtue, its inhabitants lacking this [i.e., virtue], and evil reigning, what could the good people expect except the just punishment of God for so many sins?

In this villa the fiesta of Carnival (as I have said in other parts of this *History*) has always been celebrated very much against propriety in every way, but much more so in this year [of 1719], which ended up provoking divine justice. The youth of Spain (here called *chapetones* when only recently arrived) typically find the lost women who inhabit this city to be quite easy, and thus they quickly proceed to commit many dishonest acts that cannot be declared, and if this occurs in the little festivals that fill the year, it is much more so during Carnival. They called together certain young women (although beautiful, quite insolent) as if in the court of England (when don José de la Quintana went to the merchant ships to trade for clothing, and bringing cloth to this realm they brought Englishmen) a certain heresiarch prince summoned them to dine. And with that honest gentleman [Quintana] at their table, there entered to serve the dishes six extremely beautiful unclothed damsels, stark naked, and as many young men in the same manner, and with the tablecloths torn away the twelve of them danced and left.

Women are curious in the extreme, and thus these lost women [of Potosí] determined to imitate those ones, and in order to do so the young [Spanish] men first loaded them up with aguardiente, with which they dared to drop their clothes and dance in that way, in which it is clear (all of them provoked to this great infamy) they added in others. And what happened next? The mortal epidemic sent them all to the grave so that the earth could cover up such dishonesty.[8]

---

8. This episode seems to have upset Arzáns so much that he had trouble explaining it. Apparently a Potosí merchant, Quintana, dined with English merchants in Buenos Aires, witnessed a scandalous dance, and reported it upon returning to Potosí, where locals copied it.

With all this, how could divine justice not be provoked to the point of executing a general punishment? If the indecorous and profane clothing of the body is, as Saint Augustine says, the messenger of the adulterer at heart, what of total nudity? The woman who pretends to be beautiful and resplendent before the world cannot have a chaste heart in the eyes of God. Yet, not satisfied with this apparatus, they invent new ways of revealing the neck, and now with the French fashion it is not only the neck but down to the stomach, with which it is certain that in all the world there is dishonesty in this sex. But I do not speak of everyone, as in all parts there are extremely honest women, as their status requires it, and their virtue maintains them in that most necessary perfection. I speak of the lost women who abound more in some parts than in others for the perdition of souls. Clearly there are such outfits and customs reproved by God, shameful to that sex, offensive to nature, and scandalous to civil and political decency. Really, what is more dangerous than revealing the parts that nature and honesty would cover? As for those who reveal their breasts, says the prophet [Jeremiah] in his lamentation number 4, they are the breasts of the lamias [female monsters] that do not serve except to feed the impurity of their lovers and maintain lust. What then can be said for revealing other indecencies? The woman who would reveal and make public that which ought to be hidden will someday be made to hide that which necessarily ought to be revealed.

With various types of misdeeds, the sinners of this villa finally provoked divine justice to the point of being punished, although with great mercy compared to what their sins deserved. At the beginning of this year, certain men (who were, without doubt, foreign heretics who came in great numbers from the merchant ships, as everything was uncontrolled) spoke to a little Indian boy, who spoke Spanish, and they told him that, upon taking communion one day, he should take the host from his mouth and bring it to them, that they would give him twenty pesos, and they advanced him five. He went and received communion, and, at the moment of taking it, it went down to his chest briefly (as he later declared), and then it freed itself to be taken [perhaps it magically popped back into his mouth?]. This boy went to a priest and explained the whole thing, and [the priest] said he told him to identify those Jews (as he called them) and to go back to his house, but the boy never returned nor could he ever find out more about him, and he only had word, albeit hearsay, that he had died in Tarapaya [a nearby village] while fleeing to Oruro. With such disrespect to the Divine Majesty, what could be expected?[9] Another act of disobedience preceded this punishment, which was the scandalous resistance of certain Spanish merchants to taking up the standard in the procession of Our Lady of Solitude on Holy Friday, and one of them was already obligated, as he had drawn the lot. In spite of his resistance, with a final threat he paid the cost of candle wax so that another would take up the standard, and, as God sees intentions, he decided not to permit the procession, such that before they set out he sent a great deluge of water that did not let up until the whole thing was undone. Although they tried to reach the main church (first station and near La Merced) with the holy sepulcher, they could not proceed, and they added another disrespectful act, breaking up both the ecclesiastical and secular accompaniment of the Lord, or rather his image, such that several poor men had to return the sepulcher with great indecency, when up until that time it was carried on the shoulders of the priests of the illustrious assembly (according to laudable custom). It was not a novelty that God, along with his Most Holy Mother, did not permit this procession to go forward, due to other forms of resistance and lack of devotion, as I have noted in other parts of this *History*. But this one occurred just as the plague hit.

Let us shift now to the natural causes that conjoined to create this plague, the first being God. It was already known since before the beginning of this year that one of the ships of war and trade that just reached Buenos Aires brought the plague from Europe, and, unlading in that port, it killed up to four thousand people within and outside its limits, and from there, carried by greed, it went to the Kingdom of Chile and wrought the same destruction, and from Buenos Aires it traveled to the provinces of Tucumán, Paraguay, Corrientes, and the missions of the Jesuit fathers. From there divine justice sent it directly to this villa, leaving some towns in Tucumán untouched, although later it went back to them to strike and destroy their inhabitants with innumerable mortality.

In the middle of March it began to hit this villa, no one knowing at first that it was a contagious disease, and among the first to die were the city council member don Salvador Pallares, a gentleman of

9. This story refers to the Miracle of the Profaned Host, an anti-Semitic libel.

good credit; his wife; and many children and extended family. Thus began [to fill] the sea of tears, and soon these deaths were forgotten. Never has there been seen in this kingdom nor in all those of this South America, nor, as I understand, in the northern one of New Spain, a similar contagious plague that was so widespread and durable. Typhus, chest pains, and other known ills are common enough, and in this villa, when they take hold, a lot of people tend to die, and for this reason they call these illnesses plagues, and in the same way other symptoms, like malignant fevers, intestinal blockages, diarrhea, pustules, and so on, which, adding up, they afterward give the name "plague," but as for this one there was never any precedent in all the time that the Spaniards possessed these Indies.

They [i.e., these kingdoms] have remained free of those plagues of Europe, Africa, and Asia, in which there die not thousands but millions of people: only the plague of smallpox tends to destroy the Christian and infidel Indians along with children, and even this was not seen in these kingdoms before a Black slave belonging to the marquis don Francisco Pizarro [Peru's most famous conquistador] brought it when he came with the conquest, and once it caught among the infidels it killed thousands upon thousands of them, leaving [the Spanish] in charge. For [these kingdoms] never having experienced similar plagues, it made this one [of 1719] all the more frightening, as it was an unknown and variable illness, and this is how it was described by don Matías Ciriaco y Selda, a well-accredited scientific physician, a Peruvian [Creole] from Lima, now clerical presbyter and priest of the benefice in Saint Lawrence in the city of La Plata, whose words are the following:

"The epidemic that in this villa has hit the poor with such lamentable destruction has caused such confusion among all because of the terrible and various forms with which it strikes, unlike the annual illnesses that in other years are suffered in this winter season. This one has as principal and universal agent a strange dryness (influenced by Saturn) that is drawn from the air into the blood, and being thus altered the greater part of it turns to choler, filling up the bladder receptacle with this hot and dry humor, and that which flows anew regurgitates into the most principal parts, already separated from the blood, giving rise to pains in the head and fainting spells, bitterness in

the mouth, rough spots on the back of the throat, and it tints
the face the color of citrine and especially the 'tunic' that they
call the cornea of the eyes; the urine is colored saffron, [and
there are] pains in the kidneys and loins; nausea or motions
in the stomach to try to vomit; the pulse raised, irregular, or
hidden; great dryness in the nose; a dry cough. It is the same
epidemic [disease] that struck in 1557 and 1580, killing many
'neumasinos' [apparently a word for Native Americans] so
cruel and fierce that many died on the fourth day, others the
fifth, and a few were permitted to live on to a seventh day. The
neumasinos called it coqueluchi [cocoliztli, which decimated
Mexico in the 1570s], and it brought on the same symptoms as
the present one."

    This doctor went on with the prescription that his experience
helped him to discover, but it was of use to only very few, as the just
punishment of God was already underway. If the bleedings [of the
arm] helped kill off the first ones, later those [bleedings] of the ankle
took their toll. Those who looked after some killed off others. Some
were stricken with a terrible frenzy, others with a sad melancholy,
and others with a mortal rage, and with these various symptoms
there was no relief except to die.

    This same pestilence was experienced universally in the year 1348
in the three parts of the world, and it lasted three full years, the start
of it (according to Dr. Gonzalo de Illescas in volume 2 of his *Pontifical History* in the life of Clement VI, chapter 4) was a great earthquake felt in many parts and especially in Venice, as [Marco Antonio]
Sabellico says, which lasted fifteen full days, causing all pregnant
women to miscarry. "It is an incredible thing," Illescas goes on, "that
which diverse authors say about this pestilence. Some say it began
with diarrhea and then later appeared with different symptoms." The
same occurred in this villa. "But the one I believe most," says this
author, "is Giovanni Boccaccio, who, as eyewitness, said it started in
the Orient some years before, and that at first, just having a minor
nosebleed of two or three drops, one died soon after with no remedy whatsoever."[10] The same was experienced in this villa, the only
difference being that it was not only two or three drops but gushes

10. Boccaccio is the author of the *Decameron*.

of blood, and thus they died. He goes on to say, "But after it passed here into Europe, people started to grow nodules in the groin or in the armpit, as big as apples or at least eggs. Afterward similar nodules appeared on various parts of the body." In the same way in this villa there appeared on many people pustules and sores that shortened lives. "Soon after the sickness changed," the author continues, "in the form of black or green stains (like what we here call typhus or yaws [pintas]), which appeared on the arms and legs, and within two or three days the most affected died without redemption and most of them without any fever whatsoever, nor any other symptom." Here [in Potosí] none of them lacked a terrible fever. "The sickness was so contagious that simply touching a sick person would infect you." Here not only touching clothing but merely looking at a sick person [could kill you]. And he affirms that "in only four months (March, April, May, and June) there died in Florence alone ninety-six thousand people, so many that there was no way for the churches to accommodate them." Here [in Potosí] neither the churches nor the cemeteries [could accommodate the corpses]. "It was a common occurrence," he says, "for priests to go out with one body from one house, and by the time they reached the church they had eight or nine [cadavers] that joined along the way, the citizens carrying them in procession." Francesco Petrarch (who also saw it) said that in Italy many places were so depopulated that not a living soul could be found. And in those places least hard hit, nine of ten died." In this villa it often happened that in the Indian barrios not a single rational being of the twenty or thirty formerly housed together remained alive; not even the animals remained, and in the hinterland [of Potosí] the Indian pueblos were so devastated that some had only five or ten persons remaining. "The people went out," those authors say, "to live in the countryside to flee the death striking the towns, and not only people abandoned cities but also chickens, dogs, cats, and other domestic animals, fleeing from the company of man, and all fled to the deserts, and there everyone died of plague or hunger, [beasts and] owners. They did not understand what to do," the authors go on, "except to carry out processions and perform other pious works to placate the ire of the Lord." Here [in Potosí] they performed twenty processions, as will be seen, and thirty-three public orations. Finally, if that plague in three years killed a third part of humanity (as Petronius says), within this villa alone there died over twenty-two thousand people, as will be seen later on, which in such a thinly populated kingdom (so much so that it appears a desert) is an extremely high number. To count all those who died in the space of five hundred leagues between Buenos Aires and this villa and in its twelve parishes plus the towns around it, we shall sum up later, and in all it was a most notable pity.

Also accompanying this plague was the bad influence of the stars that presided over this year 1719, for which reason was seen such great despoliation in this villa. Saturn and Mars were in opposition, very noxious for the human temperament, which, as experience shows, they kill those who look at them with homicidal rays if not mitigated by other lights or these among themselves, like the two poisons that a poet hails: *pina venena*, etc. (which the curious reader will have already seen in the judgment of this year); they do not temper their damages, the fire of Mars [un]moderated by the ice of Saturn. A witness to this was the malignant color of their splendor, one leaden and the other brazen, indicating the nature of their bodies.

This year (both placed in our Southern Hemisphere, near the two points of the ellipses that pass along our zenith in the opposed signs of Scorpio and Aquarius), it was clear that we would be infected, but mostly because of Mars, which in addition to this was found to be at its nearest point to earth and to the east, qualities that with others gave it dominion over the year, and in addition the two eclipses of moon and sun that in this year were visible to us, the moon on the fifth of March and the sun on August 15, which were so damaging, especially in this villa, where, although Jupiter and Mercury predominated and its [i.e., Potosí's] signs are Gemini and Libra (as I have said at the start of this *History*, along with that which they influence), of the seven vertical stars that pass over it, five of them (which are the Eye of the Crow, which Copernicus called the collar or back of the neck; and the Austrina star facing Scorpio [Corona Australis]; and the one at the outer edge of the arc of Sagittarius; and the one behind the head of Sagittarius; and the one right after it), all five are of the nature of Mars, and those in Sagittarius and Scorpio, which prompt only wars, dissentions, hatreds, disputes, deaths, and injuries, as I have already said, and the other two stars, that of the right leg of the dragon [sic] Ofiuchus is of the nature of Venus, and the southern antecedent of the spine of Capricorn is of the nature of Mercury, trade and commerce, venereal occupations, and so on, but all this is stated in its place.

Thus, then, given the principal role that this malignant planet [Mars] has in its path, having the referred precedence and combining with everything else, brought forth the terrible destruction that we experienced. And to continue describing it we shall need another chapter, saying in concluding this one that in the beginning of the month of March (which is when, as I have said, the plague began), there reached this villa the news of the breaking of the peace between England and Spain and the unjust rout the English visited on the Spanish navy returning from the rescue of Sicily. And thus it was known that all goods and capital belonging to the English in Cádiz, Panama, Cartagena, Buenos Aires, and this villa were confiscated, the news followed by the order of general don Manuel de Villavicencio y Granada [corregidor, or governor of Potosí], seizing 60,000 pesos proceeding from the sales of [enslaved] Blacks they brought from Buenos Aires.

Also the Basques who were in this villa received no small grief and worry in hearing news of the civil disturbances taking place in their country, which, as everyone knows, were over customs duties. It was about the time when don José de la Quintana was setting out for Buenos Aires with his brother (a cleric who was already ordained as a preacher) plus don Miguel de Zubiegui, don Gregorio de Otálora, and others of this singular nation, with 3 million [pesos] in silver and other riches to take to Spain. God had promised them a safe voyage, to keep them from running into the many enemies they feared they might encounter, as they no doubt awaited them at sea, although (as I have already said) they left this villa wrung out [i.e., broke, penniless], unprepared for great trials with the plague already inside its walls.


Chapter XLVII

Continuing with the mortality of the plague and the many processions and public orations they performed, to which heaven responded with the same indifference.

Death by sin is so cruel that, if the sinner really understood, it would be a lot cheaper to die a thousand deaths of the body than only one by sin. Ah, villa of Potosí! What a state you're in! Your neglect of God was so great that it brought you to a state in which God could not hear your pleas, that He could not see the tears of the good inhabitants, seeking mercy for themselves and for the evil as well. How could such love for earthly things end, the injustices laid bare before your very eyes; the disturbances and disputes in every street, plaza, or house; the unbridled acts of turpitude; the repeated sacrileges; all manner of sins given free rein, how could it all end except in a thousand laments and in so many accelerated deaths?

That's how it was, then, upon entering the month of April, one began to see each day buried ten, twelve, and more bodies, especially of the Indians and the poor, as among those unfortunate Natives [the plague] was unleashed with fury, continuing to the point of annihilating them. This villa was already alarmed and everyone afraid, although many of the rich made light of it at first, as there were not so many bodies per day, but soon the number of deaths rose. The good and the bad remained confident that the Lord would always have pity after public prayers, and thus there began various novenas, as they did in the monastery of Saint Dominic, first to the Peruvian Saint Rose of Saint Mary [of Lima], patron of this villa. In the parish of Saint Bernard [they prayed] to Saint Thomas Aquinas. In that of Saint Roch of [the barrio of] El Tío to this saint, patron and advocate against plague, and the same was done in [the parish of] Saint Roch of Vilasirca and in the Convent of the Remedies to their [i.e., the nuns'] spouse, Christ our Lord.

Beginning in this month of April, His Majesty's ministers suspended the rents of the Carmelite nuns of Saint Theresa in this city, according to a decree mandating that all royal rents be withheld for four years for the use of His Majesty. And, being brides of the Lord, they had their rents impounded based on 72,000 pesos kept in the royal mint, whose monthly yield was 300 pesos, and [the money] being withheld from them during that time, they had to live at the mercy of the townsfolk to survive, as there was no other means available, although they searched the records. There came to their assistance the noble householders (sharing the burden), maintaining [the nuns] with great compassion, seeing what great tribulations fell on these servants of the Lord, whose laments and tears were certainly enough to break hearts.

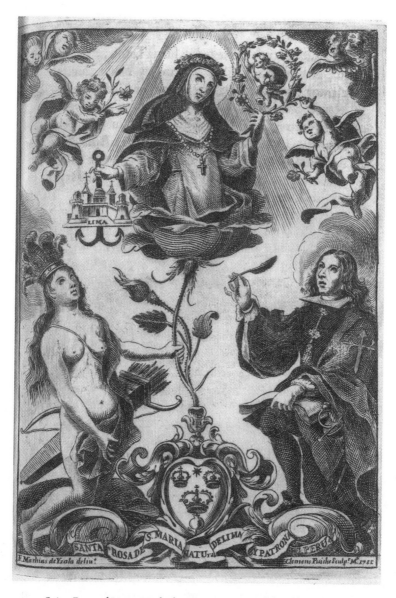

FIG. 5. Saint Rose of Lima, Madrid, 1711. Courtesy of the John Carter Brown Library at Brown University, Providence, RI.

Thanks to this and other good works, the Divine Majesty permitted that the disaster we shall refer to was not so generalized as to finish off this villa outright. Virtue is affable by nature, and thus by nature abhorrent the fault, and the strange thing is that although there are vicious people practicing virtues, no virtuous people practice vices. There were bad and good in this villa. What would have happened to it had there not been more good than simply bad? With their evil deeds these [bad] ones provoked divine justice, but with the good, the others merited some mercy.

Friday, April 28, seeing the destruction being wrought by the plague, by disposition of the town council and ecclesiastical authorities, they carried to the church of Saint Dominic all the images of the patrons of this villa, so as to go from there in procession to the main church, where a public prayer and supplication began so that these patron saints might intercede with the Lord so as to mitigate his rigor. And in the procession there went Saint Augustine, Saint Francis Xavier, Saint Sebastian, Saint Roch, Saint Barbara, and Saint Rose, and, beginning on Saturday the twenty-ninth, the secular clergy commenced with their sung mass and supplication, and later there followed the regular clergy until Sunday, May 7, on which day they made a most devout procession to all the churches along the most principal streets, pleading with God for mercy, which the whole villa attended, accompanying their patron saints, and throughout these nine days all the city's church bells tolled.

The most noble town council and its most noble head did not miss any of these incessant functions, with supplications going on morning and evening, sermons, masses, public prayers, and processions with great devotion, setting a notable example for the whole town, not escaping any discomforts or the rigorous cold weather and other celestial disturbances, paying for certain novenas, persuading and encouraging others and performing other pious works that will be detailed later. Oh, how good the example of the leaders, the nobles, the powerful can be so that virtue may be esteemed, as the authority of such personages tears off the masks introduced by vanity and self-love to make ugly and despicable the yearning for perfection.

In this procession of the patron saints, they brought out the Holy Christ from the chapel of the Blessed Souls of Purgatory, which is most devout, its confraternity being, as I have said elsewhere, in the main church, that since the ruin of the Lima earthquake [of 1687] (which in its place I described) had not been brought out. There accompanied this devout procession all the venerable clergy and priests, members of the religious orders, the nobility, and the common folk. The main church's image of the [Immaculate] Conception, dressed in purple, went out in this procession, accompanied by all of the feminine sex, and throughout the procession there were in attendance innumerable souls with great affliction and tears.

Before this procession (which was Wednesday, May 3), there was one for Saint Rose, following a sermon preached in the monastery of Saint Dominic by the very reverend father Fray Juan de Águilar, apostolic preacher whom we mentioned in the previous chapter, who preached with his accustomed and fervent spirit and tenderness.

Monday, eighth of May, following the day of the procession of the patron saints, there commenced another most devout novena of supplication in [the church of] Saint Francis to the Holy Christ of the True Cross, unique refuge from the trials of this villa, and to Saint Francis of Assisi and to Saint Francis Solano, a saint who in his lifetime was in this villa, as we have stated in its place in this *History*.

Thursday, eleventh of May, in the midst of the novena for this miraculous Lord, there began another to the father of the poor, Saint John of God, in his church, and on Tuesday, May 16, they carried out the "blood procession" of the Holy Christ of the True Cross, with which they ended their supplication by way of the [several] "Saint Francises," and there went out as well the [procession of the] patriarch Saint Joseph and the Mother of God of Solitude, which was most devout and penitent, in which for being so (because when the Lord of the True Cross goes out, Potosí ordinarily empties entirely into the streets to accompany him; it was more so on this occasion when the divine justice was so irritated by sins) and thus accompanying all this were the nobility and the common people, innumerable souls and women marching alongside with huge candles in large numbers. This procession went out at four in the afternoon after a sermon preached by the very reverend father Fray Juan de Relúz, and it finished at eight at night.

The devotion to this Lord of the True Cross and many of his miracles are recorded in the course of this *History*. It has been portentous and permanent. He has held the affection of the whole town, so much so that in the 174 years that have passed since its 1545 foundation, minus the 4 that passed from the discovery of the Cerro Rico

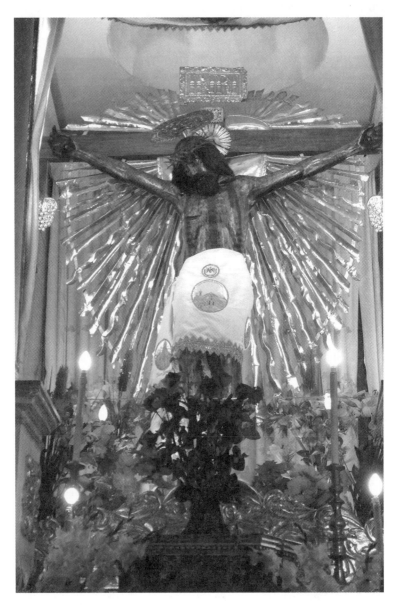

FIG. 6. Holy Christ of the True Cross, Potosí. Photo by the author.

until this cult was introduced with the appearance of this prodigious image, as noted in its place), in these 170 years leading up to this one of 1719, according to the books and good computations, they have given in alms 2,020,000 pesos, and in most of the early years alms surpassed 12,000 pesos, just to display the devotion and greatness of this villa. And in the same way and in 174 years that have passed since they started the cult of the Souls [of Purgatory] and shortly thereafter its sodality, which had its origin in the parish of Saint Lawrence, which was then the villa's main church, its inhabitants have given 3,336,000 pesos in alms, because all told in alms they ingathered 400 pesos per week, likely more than less, which adds up to this sum.

Friday, May 19, the procession of Saint John of God was performed at the end of his novena, and in the same went the image of Saint Raphael and that of the miraculous Saint John of God of the infirmary, for which not a day passes that they do not experience God's marvels by its intercession and more so among the sick of that hospital where he has been visibly seen taking care of them many times. They also brought out for this procession the image of the Mother of God of Carmen, whose making and marvels I have already noted, and the whole of this villa accompanied her.

Easter Monday of the Holy Spirit, which was the twenty-ninth of May, the dawn having revealed 10 bodies of the poor at the doors of the Charity Hospital and around town another 20 dead, the pains of those alive grew, and they knew not what to do with themselves, as in less than sixty days there had perished more than 2,500 people, 2,140 of them Indians and the rest poor Spaniards of this villa, along with mestizos and outsiders, but only 2 or 3 rich persons. And, although the majority of the dead were Indians, the pain was no less, as without them the villa is but a body without feet or hands. Whole dwellings were emptied of these unfortunate folk. Even the dogs (which many raise) all perished, and the worst of it was that the plague had not even taken hold as it soon would, beginning in the month of June. This fatal illness took hold of this accursed villa with [a total population of] 60,000 people, between both sexes, all nations, statuses, and ages, a small number compared with how many it maintained in other times [ca. 120,000 in 1620].

Before going on with the supplications and processions, I shall start by referring to some of the memorable cases that were deemed peculiar to this destruction done by God's justice, irritated by sins. I shall not relate all of them, as for that one would need a separate treatise. The venerable Jesuit fathers, among those who worked incessantly to such great effect for souls during this plague, wrote a treatise of many folios, which they sent off to their head officer in Rome with the father procurators of this kingdom, who at the time were about to leave for Europe, and despite not being even half the annual letter of 1719, there having passed only five months since the disaster hit, its volume was huge. What sort of things had they experienced as confessors of so many dying? One day it will come to light (should God be served) to provide special examples.

I write in these brief chapters only that which happened to become known among some of the living, and I leave out their names, as that seems proper. That which I would most like to inscribe on paper, bronze, and stone is the incomparable charity with which these venerable [Jesuit] fathers treated the dying, paying no attention to the terrible contagion from which they might perish, as it was such that not even children, spouses, and parents wanted to get close to the sick unless they had to, and later it stuck to them and they all died, and God sought to reward such perfect charity, as these Jesuits displayed such that none of them was touched by the plague.

They all set out from the shelter of their college and barely returned for a snack before going back to other sick ones, some on foot and others in pairs on horseback to [visit] those outside town, in sun, cold, and other rigors of weather until late at night, with incredible fatigue but greater charity, patiently snatching souls from the devil's jaws, in which they experienced frightening successes, especially with Father Tomás Rodríguez, procurator of Castile, a man of admirable virtue and spiritual father of this whole villa, mediator of all evil and qualified consultant of all that pertains to soul and body. All, in the end, from top to bottom (if such a great company could have an inferior) labored in this disaster, and, by the time they sent their accounts to Rome, there had accumulated more than ten thousand declarations that they alone had given the viaticum [final sacrament], and later they added many to this number.

In the same way I would like to emphasize the great charity of the Bethlehemite fathers, as in their general hospital they practiced the greatest charity with bodies and souls of so many ill, such that in most months they labored over 250 patients, the cost of bread alone being impossible to cover, at ten or twelve pesos per day. And what would the cost of other supplies and medicines have been, when by trusted account it would have been a [silver] piece of eight per patient per day? The most burdensome thing was that all the service people perished with the contagion, and the fathers themselves took to carrying the dying, taking them to their sepulchers, anointing them, and all the rest, as no one can deny, from which some of these religious were hit with the plague, and it was divine providence that they did not all perish, although some did, but most escaped. Only in Saint John of God, not being a general hospital, did the father-nurses die along with others who tended them, such that there remained only the prelate, although even he missed nothing in his every obligation.[11] Let us now move on to refer to one of the exemplary events that occurred during this disaster.

Only so as not to see women when they are certain to be the instrument of their perdition might men wish to be born blind. What great damages have resulted from gazing on them! They are enemies of the soul, the eyes, servants who let the thief into the house. Female beauty is an enchantment that wordlessly seizes all understanding and silently persuades the will to captivity and from there to perdition.

There lived in this villa a noble youth, so struck and bound at first sight by the beauty of a certain damsel, his neighbor, that, in following his lustful appetite, he enjoyed her for the space of four years, giving great grief to his mother, a widow, and to two damsel sisters he had, all three pleading with him incessantly to cease this offense against God. This had no effect, and he even mocked their counsels, and the lamentations rose, with which God sent the final warning by way of the contagion he caught from turpitude with that female companion, who also later died. His virtuous mother, seeing that he was in imminent danger of death, called on two learned and virtuous priests with tears in her eyes that they might help in that critical moment.

They did just that, and upon his having received all the sacraments, one day at the end of the month of May, his mother was called on to give him her blessing. She gave it and returned to her house so as not to see him die with her own eyes, as he later died.

---

11. The church of the Brothers Hospitallers of Saint John of God included an infirmary.

The priests then went to the afflicted mother to console her, telling her how he had died with many signs of repentance, and that without doubt his soul was in a good state, and that the last thing he did was to suddenly recover his strength, and, as they were seated, he got up out of the bed with incredible speed and, jumping over to the wall before him, he clapped it twice with the palm of his hand, saying, "María! María!" And returning to his bed with the same speed, at that moment he fell dead.

Upon hearing these final words, his pious mother gave out a great shriek and leaped to her feet, saying, "Ay, my lords, my son is condemned, since in such an extreme moment he called on his paramour, who yet lives and has her room behind that same wall that he struck. Her name is María, and by this word alone he called her." This alarmed the priests, and, not being able to do anything else, as nothing at all could console the mother, they left that house. Within an hour that woman who had called them lay dead, not even having received a single sacrament, as she had lost track of time and had forgotten to request them for the five full days that had passed since the symptoms began. The state of their souls only God knows.

The fire with which the star of Mars burned was already so frightening in this month of May that seeing it to the east, where it appeared, caused dizzy spells and aches in the head and eyes. It was like a very lively and great fire to see, and thus the fury of the plague epidemic was such that it seemed not one living person left in this villa would survive. And with this fear the supplications did not cease, and on Easter Monday of the Holy Spirit, which was May 29, there commenced from [the monastery of] Saint Augustine another novena to the Christ of Burgos and to his Most Holy Mother of Copacabana, to Saint Nicholas Tolentino, Saint John of Sahagún, and Saint Rita, in which the very reverend father Fray Francisco Romero, apostolic missionary, had them announce an indulgence-filled mission jubilee, and he preached every day like the most admirable preacher he was (as has been said in this *History*), reminding every-one of the warnings that God, justly angered by the sins of this villa, had announced by way of earlier missions, and they performed a devout procession on Tuesday with innumerable accompaniment and many candles of the devout, as will be seen later on.

Tuesday, May 30, there began the annual novena for Christ of the Column, from [the monastery of] La Merced, which also tended to the plague. The sermon that started it was as fervent as it was tender, as it was noted that never had it been seen that the dogs ate the cadavers as soon as death came, which happened in the barrios and townships of the parish of San Pedro and other places, as the poor Indians were so numerous and here and there every one of them dead. They performed this novena for Christ of the Column, for the miraculous image of Our Lady of Solitude, and for Saint Peter Nolasco. At the same time they performed a supplication in the parish of Saint Lawrence to the miraculous Holy Christ, who, as I mentioned elsewhere in this *History*, spoke to his priest don Francisco Aguirre, converting him by his sacred fear. Another novena was performed at the same time to the most adored and miraculous crucified Christ of the parish of San Pedro.

On the fourth of June, a Sunday, a procession went out from [the monastery of] La Merced and in it the Christ of the Column (now thirty-two years having passed since it went out in another procession when Lima was ruined by an earthquake), the Mother of God of Solitude, and Saint Peter Nolasco. The whole villa accompanied them with many candles, having preached beforehand the reverend father Fray Nicolás de la Rosa, of this redemptionist order [of the Mercedarians] with clear doctrine.

On the next day, the fifth of June, the procession set out after the reverend father Fray Juan de Águilar, apostolic preacher, held forth in the parish of San Pedro with his customary fervent doctrine. He walked alongside through all the streets of this parish and others in this villa, accompanied by a great portion of the folk with many candles, Spaniards and Indians with the Holy Christ, which I've already said is their miraculous image, and also the miraculous image of the [Virgin of] Candlemas (which we have already noted in this *History*) and Saint Vincent Ferrer [Valencian patron of orphans], Saint Rose, Saint Peter, and Saint Paul. Hearts broke in this procession with the pain of seeing so many little Indian girls of four, five, or six years of age, many of them orphans, their parents having died in this plague, some naked and others with funeral tunics, weighed down with crosses and crowns of thorns on their heads.

Tuesday, the sixth of June, the procession of the Holy Christ of Burgos went out with images of the Mother of God and the previously named saints, right after the reverend missionary father preached eight days of mission, and, as this last one finished, he performed the *vía sacra* through the churches where the procession stopped, and in the streets he went discharging arrows of words. There accompanied this procession innumerable men and women with many candles.

Thursday, the eighth of June, day of Corpus [Christi], there began another novena in the Jesuit compound to the Holy Eucharist, to his Most Holy Mother, and to my Lady Saint Ann, and to Saint Joachim, and the next day another supplication before the Eucharist in the main church, but the plague only spread right after each supplication.

One must greatly praise the kindness and acclaim the charity of Dr. don José de la Piedra, new priest of the parish of Saint Roch of El Tío, as so many bodies of the poor were cast in front of the chapel of Our Lady of La Misericorcia of the Indians, and many were from other curates that (for fear that they would not have sufficient payment before the others died of hunger) they dropped them there, and alongside the poor of the parish of Saint Roch this pious man buried them, carrying them from the main plaza, where this chapel is, to Saint Roch, which is many blocks away. The bodies were carried and accompanied by the Indian Confraternity of La Misericordia, founded in that parish. And during the time that the plague lasted, these poor ones buried in their cemetery over two thousand bodies, which this good priest personally oversaw. When the holy fear of God guards the house of the conscience, the common enemy with his batteries cannot break in. Where there is discretion, kindness, and mercy, there is no space for tyranny, deception, or cruelty. So much of this has been felt in this kingdom.

Saturday, June 17, seeing the worsening of the plague, the devout Spaniards began another novena to the Holy Christ of the parish of Saint Lawrence, to the miraculous image of the Candlemas of Jerusalem, to the patriarch Saint Joseph, and to Saint Lawrence and Saint Sebastian, and they ended with a very devout procession, which the whole villa accompanied, and on few occasions or maybe never before had these two miraculous images of Christ and his Most Holy Mother gone out together.

The most lamentable thing amid this whole tribulation was that due to the great poverty that the poor suffered (Indians as well as Spaniards), they died, and it so happened that those who took care of the rich as much as possible cured them, and there was no one left to care for those poor folks, particularly those who could have done so. These ones said they had nothing to offer the poor, and yet they did not lack for their gambling addictions, as they began the night at the gaming tables and were still there at dawn, and they lacked nothing for the delicacies of the plate, for the vanities of clothing, for household furnishings, for a multitude of servants, for the costs of pretension and lawsuits, for the bribes of ambition, for the furnaces of Babylon, for the caves of turpitude, for the houses of Delilah and Rahab that Saint Augustine called the houses of hell. For all this they feared they would not have enough, and thus they did not rescue the poor from extreme necessity, in whose grip they rendered their lives.

Another novena was carried out in the chapel of the Mount of Calvary at the same time that the one was performed in Saint Lawrence, and it was to Christ our Savior with the cross on his shoulders, which is their most adored image, and the procession passed with measured accompaniment and candles.

At this time the illustrious sodality of Our Lady of La Misericordia of the Spaniards (about whom I have spoken in various parts of this *History*) occupied themselves in collecting the bodies of so many poor that it greatly fatigued them, as there were so many (some 10, 14, 18, or more each day) and also for all the decay that had occurred in most, and they brought them to the chapel of the main plaza, horrifying this whole villa, and there Dr. Francisco Montoya, helper of priests, with total decency and accompaniment of the confraternity and many illustrious persons, buried them in the church of La Misericordia, and after this [church] filled with bodies they did the same in the old church of this vocation and then in the cemetery, until there was no more space in these churches, and to end the horror of the main plaza they took them to [the parish church of] Saint Martin, as will later be seen, after having buried 1,500 poor persons. It was most notable the charity of Dr. Montoya and of the brotherhood of La Misericordia, and thus God permitted that in recompense not one of them was touched by this contagion. And when has charity not received such rewards? Thus piety should never be scarce, as it is quickly rewarded for its deeds.

There were others not lacking in charity amid this immense evil that fell on this villa, and among them was the general don Silvestre de Briñas, of the Order of Santiago, who came to the point of dispensing with his own hands the medicines, ointments, and clysters for the poor Indians, sending them victuals and other necessary

things, up until the time when he had to leave this villa. He who
sees God in the poor and relieves them, in each one he searches for a
chaplain to beg for him, and the Lord himself, as the one served, gives
from the piety that is shown to them, as he loves them so much, he
multiplies the capital so that he would have more to give them with
which to succor them, remaining on the road but obliged to return
with immense rewards of glory.

The plague did great damage, but poverty did more because the
symptoms required sweats, enemas, and herbs to correct the choler
(and because they totally lost their desire to eat), and the poor did not
even have beds to lie on while sweating but only a blanket or an old
rag, nor anyone nor any way to administer the enemas, nor anything
whatsoever to eat, and thus, for the poor one who fell ill, the only
remedy was death.

In the early days of June, a call went out from a house to a priest,
a cleric who passed by in the street. He entered to see what was
wanted, and he found two sick girls in a small dwelling that seemed
more like a rabbit warren than a human habitation, lying on a cow-
hide with no more covering than their skirts and shawls. The symptoms had fiercely taken hold of both of them. They were beautiful,
although now disfigured, and so honest that from afar one could
see their virginal state. They asked the priest to confess them so as
to receive the viaticum, but he found himself confused due to the
narrowness of the bed and the room, yet they recognized him and
said they were sisters and damsels and that, since their mother had
died of the same illness twenty days before, and having no relatives
besides a single female cousin, whom they had no means of contact-
ing to explain their situation, they found themselves in that state due
to poverty. Touched, the priest confessed them as best he could, and
together they asked that, with the permission of the curate, they be
brought the viaticum and holy oils and that he alone plus the sexton
should enter, as he had already seen them shirtless. The priest, full
of sorrow, left for the curate or his assistant, and in his company he
returned with the holy sacraments, and as they had requested he
administered them. The men left them some alms, and later the priest
brought them some shirts and two blankets, food, and some medicines, with which divine will and this charity freed them from that
danger, and today they are found serving God. And if only they had
had this aid many others would have escaped.

On June 22 there began another novena of supplication in Santo Domingo to Our Lady of the Rosary, to the holy patriarchs Saint Dominic, Saint Francis, Saint Vincent Ferrer, and Saint Hyacinth. They performed this novena with the same confidence that, in this same year at the end of January, they had performed that novena I mentioned of this most beautiful image of the [Virgin of the] Rosary for the great rains that ruined the buildings, and at that point they ceased. At the end of this [month], the procession followed a sermon, which was Sunday, July 2, with the whole villa going out in accompaniment. Yet what followed was greater mortality, as [the disease] gripped harder as winter came on (which in our hemisphere is June 22), and it now struck the Spanish folk and illustrious families, as the sins of many were rising, without fear of God or of death.

That is what happened, then, on the day of Saint John, the good folk performing the supplication of Our Lady of the Rosary, which, as I have said, began on June 22. There gathered in a certain house to celebrate the day of a certain foreign woman (perdition of souls in this villa) eleven men and nine women, and they set to dancing that night that damned *son* that at the same time they sing and dance, which in the language of the Indians they call *Caymari vida*, which is the chorus, and in Castilian it is the same as saying, "This is living; this is fun," quite similar to the Spanish *chacona* and its *zarabanda* so popular among the vulgar youth. It being, then, ten at night, and there having preceded various dishonesties, some sang as others danced with that refrain of "This is the life," when (a strange occurrence) they heard a very sonorous and frightening voice that came out from behind a bed, saying, "It is nothing more than death."

All those men and women were instantly filled with horror, and, as if hit with an arrow, each one fell ill with that sickness, except a certain damsel, who, with more reflection than all those other lascivious ones, got up from the remotest corner of the room, where she was, and threw herself at the feet of an image of Our Lady of the [Immaculate] Conception and cried out, "Most Holy Virgin, have pity on me, as I did not come here of my own will, but rather my aunt forced me to come," and, adding other tender pleas and promising to serve her and to serve God, she was freed, doubtless by intercession of our Lady and by her innocence. The rest [of the women] and all the men, upon returning home, died within eight days, although there escaped after three lapses a married woman who was there among the others.

Two of the men with whom I was acquainted referred to this incident when I went to see them, and I told them that [the sound] could have been a human voice, that of someone in that gathering who did this as a joke—although the scare it gave had a genuine effect. But in the moment they were in, which was the point of death without remedy, they assured me that it was a supernatural voice, as the most fearless among them searched with lamps and found no one who could have done it other than divine justice.

We human beings are so obstinate that with neither good nor ill can God get through to us. His punishments (as seen in this case and others) do not get us to mend our ways, and necessities do not soften us, but rather in the very presence of punishment the offenses against God mount, as in this case. Clay, then, is what we are; just as clay hardens under the sun's rays, the same it is with us when it comes to the favors of heaven. They do not soften us but rather harden us, and thus God sends us punishment, although in this case it was pious, as the eleven men and seven women all died with the sacraments and apparently contrite. Another novena was done in [the church of] San Benito to a miraculous image of Christ our Savior with the cross on his shoulders that is in that parish, and on July 1 they carried out a devout procession, climbing up to the main plaza.

On Sunday, July 9, there began the annual novena of the miraculous crucified Christ that they call "of the choir" and that is now located in the church of Our Lady of La Misericordia. They call it "of the choir" because, while [it was] hanging in the choir of the main church, certain infamous female witches had lit candles at one end, and the musicians entering found the fallen Lord above them, although [suspended] in the air, without getting burned, perpendicularly, and this fall occasioned by superstition was turned into exaltation of the cult of this sacred image. They carried out a devout procession to the end of the novena, in which they took out this hallowed image that had never gone outside, to the [church of] the Mother of God of La Misericordia and to Saint Francis de Paul with great accompaniment and lights.

Monday, July 10, as final refuge, [the city] being so stricken, the cost covered by the gentlemen of the town council, there began another novena to my Lady Saint Ann in the main church, to the apostle Saint Peter, and to the patriarchs Saint Joachim and Saint Joseph. On July 12, among seventeen bodies of Indians that appeared at dawn at the doors of La Misericordia [in the main plaza], there were three people asphyxiated, and they were a man, a woman, and a boy, and despite all possible inquiries they could not determine who had put them there like that, nor was there a single Indian nor Spaniard who knew who they were, which was a notably bad thing while we were experiencing the lash of divine justice for the sins of this villa. The Indian woman was pregnant, and the physicians declared that they were all strangled with two hands and some thick thing, according to what they could determine. It is not uncommon that amid such tribulations evil men are the executioners of others.

They were very notable and also wondrous the circumstances of this exemplary punishment and its terrible particulars, as among adulterers of both sexes (this being of the most public ones) more than 130 perished, many remedies proving insufficient, and only one, who valued the intercession of our father Saint Francis, escaped. Some had carried on with this type of sin for twenty years, others fifteen, others ten, some four and six, and out of all of them only this one [person] survived. It was with the same publicity and shamelessness with which they committed these adulteries that they were made known in number and circumstance, and as [adultery] is such an enormous sin, God punished it without reserve. These sinners were most forgetful of divine justice, making light of his mercy, and with the hope of forgiveness they lost their fear of punishment. They hoped for the reward and refused to give up sin, but God knows the state in which each will end.

There may have been only one consolation amid this great trial: that very few died without the sacraments, that in this the esteemed priests were not lacking, either in the main church or in the fifteen other parishes, as they usually went out in the morning to administer them, one priest from the main church or one of his assistants, without returning until midday, handing off to another assistant who would not return until seven at night, at which hour another companion would take his turn until midnight. The assistants of the parishes worked in the same way, and it was a most frightful thing to see these priests crossing the streets and plazas with the holy sacraments, always with a quick step due to the risk of illness among all. And thus they gathered to carry off a Spaniard from this street to bury, from those [streets] another, or four or ten or more, Indians, by some [streets] they carried six poor [cadavers] to the charity, by others a slave or poor Black. Everything was a horrifying confusion, and all an inconsolable sorrow that had never ever been seen in this villa. In the barrios of the parish of San Pedro, Santiago, and San Roque de Vilasirca, they came to discover many ruinous women, some who had not confessed for ten or twenty years, and, what is more, had not heard mass, as they were busy with spells and witchcraft, with diabolical pacts. Of these not one remained. All died, although most of them after repenting, in which the Jesuit fathers worked very hard. And, if a few escaped, they were of the least perverse sort, and all was mended.

Of the always at-risk youth, there were notable coincidences, as when one [young man], being on the verge of death from the epidemic, said he could see Death, all bones seated in the corner of his room, and that he pointed with his finger at a flaming bonfire that he also saw, saying that this was how life ended. Another Spanish youth who always occupied himself in lustful and dishonest behaviors said he saw four horrible forms with disembodied heads, and they threatened to place him in a frightening fiery furnace, saying they would throw him in there as soon as he expired, and upon saying this he died.

A young mestiza, who for her beauty accumulated for herself and for others many offenses against God, said that the demons were present, tearing a man apart (who had already died of the plague and had been her companion in turpitude), and that they had already placed him in one of the cauldrons of molten lead that were there nearby, and that they threatened to throw her in the other, and giving out a frightening scream she died, I being present there, helping her and exhorting her to repent.

Another who a regular [clergy] helped to die, I being present as well, said that for him there was no salvation and that he had always served the devil and that he went there to those infernos, and thus he died, his face frozen in such a horrifying expression that I almost could not lower his body from the bed. Two foreign women, invoking the names of their lovers and begging their help, expired with few signs of salvation.

Thus there occurred other frightening cases related to us by relatives of the subjects left behind, and at the least conjecture it became clear: God took mercy on all of them. Many also converted even without experiencing symptoms, leaving behind the turpitude that up until that moment they had followed to perdition. Others married their lovers, and a great many did this, although only under duress.

Tuesday, July 18, they performed a procession with my Lady Saint Ann, plus Saint Joachim, Saint Joseph, and Saint Peter, which the whole villa accompanied with many candles, and the next day, Wednesday, they did the one mentioned earlier with the Holy Christ of the Choir. Another four novenas and further supplications were performed in the nunnery of the Carmelites of Saint Theresa, and also in the convent of the nuns of Our Lady of the Remedies, and in both cases the penances and mortifications were quite grand, and extremely tender the supplications they made for the whole villa, and it was a notable thing that the brides of Christ were untouched by the contagion, especially the Carmelites, and although it did touch those of [the Convent of] the Remedies, where a nun died, plus a novice and a girl raised there, and a few female servants, it immediately ceased, and it would have been a terrible shame [otherwise], as there are more than six hundred souls in cloister.

At the end of the novena, they carried out the procession of Saint Theresa, all the villa accompanying her, and in it there went out the image of the Most Holy Mother of Carmen, Saint Theresa of Jesus, Saint Joseph, the patriarch Saint Elias, and Saint Aloysius, which was Sunday, July 23. Still the plague was in full [force], and, as a result, some men and women fled for Chuquisaca [Sucre] and other places, and, arriving there good and healthy, they died, the plague not yet being in those parts, a notable thing.

Seeing so much and such continuous mortality, the pious town council, also seeing that what most consumed the sick was their poverty, they gathered some 1,200 pesos, helped by merchants and other householders, and gave that whole amount to the charitable Jesuit fathers and to the priests of the main church so as to administer sacraments. Recognizing the poverty of each, they alleviated them with these alms. The council also decided that the physicians should attend to the poor without pay and also the pharmacies, that in receiving the prescriptions they should dispense them, obliging themselves to cover the costs. Some of the esteemed aldermen and other noble persons helped out with linen, giving so many yards so as to enshroud so many poor and also paying those who dug graves and other costs. They gave many alms to whatever brotherhood requested it, a pious work that pleased our Lord and would help satisfy guilt, as everybody knows that almsgiving is most satisfying, and, where there is true charity, there is no space for servile fear nor ignorance with either voluntary or forced poverty. There is no space for the fatal frowns of envy or ever-noxious gossip, nor is it impeded by the inquietudes of avarice. But I say again that this is when charity is true.

On August 2, after the most solemn feast that two days before they held for the patriarch Saint Ignatius, there began in his church a most devout novena and supplication to the holy remnant of the True Cross of Our Lord (the Jesuit fathers possessing a large piece of this relic), of the holy shroud touched by the one that enveloped the body of the Lord, an image of our Lady at her presentation in the temple, to the patriarch Saint Ignatius, to Saint Francis Xavier, and to the beatified Saint John Francis Régis, missionary of France.

There were preached three sermons in the course of this supplication, and, on the night of the day it began, the Lord went out through the streets to collect and convert sinners, in which were done tender acts of contrition and elegies through the streets and plazas as during mission, and on the last day, which was of Saint Lawrence, there went out in procession the relics and saints mentioned earlier, adding the Baby Jesus bearing the cross, which was accompanied by a great number of Indians, pleading with God to lift the lash of his justice. The whole villa went along, men and women accompanying it with innumerable illuminations. The clergy carried the two relics of the holy splinter and the shroud with purple surplices and stoles, all of which has never been seen in the streets of Potosí. Along went the children barefoot, in tunics, crowns [of thorns] on their heads, and bearing crosses, all of which provoked great sorrow and compunction.

Back on July 23 they had begun another supplication in the parish of San Pedro to the Eucharist and to various saints that are in that church. On August 1 they started another novena in the parish of San Sebastián to this patron saint of the villa and of the plague, and, when they took him out of the main church, the town council and its most noble leader, they placed on the saint two relics that the priest of that church had: one bone sliver of that saint and the other a splinter of the beam to which he had been tied and shot with arrows, and with this the town council (which for four years already due to dissentions and political maneuvers had not entered into its church, when for its feast they had carried him as patron, although from its doors it returned) on this occasion they were in line with the priest, and at the end of the novena the procession was finished, accompanied by the town council and the people. And for that which remains to be said about this lamentable devastation, let us open another chapter.

## Chapter XLVIII

In which continues the material of the preceding two chapters and notes also how, according to a royal decree that arrived by way of Buenos Aires from His Catholic Majesty, [we were] to receive a second time as viceroy of these kingdoms the most illustrious and most excellent lord archbishop of La Plata.

The great weight of grandeur cannot be sustained by the error of human fortune, on which it is founded. It is always negated, the solid mass of that which rises too much, dropping with greater velocity from its high point. Nature itself tends toward continuous alternation and change: all is growth and shriveling away. Rare is the time when grandeur is perpetual and durable. This villa says so with four destructions that with this one [i.e., the 1719 pandemic] it has experienced, as with the first three this *History* says as much. Various times its grandeur climbed as high as it could, and later there followed its fall. Now its luck was annihilated, caught so overwhelmed with trials and poverty. This was such (as I have already said) that it helped to take many lives, and, coming on so strong, it completely erased them, as one saw strewn in the streets the beds, clothing, and rags of the poor in the dung heaps and fields, everything thrown out, as all was contagious, and with the same desire they had in life to gain these miserable things, in death they left it all behind, and it was nothing but horror to see and touch.

They performed other supplications at the start of August to the patriarch Saint Dominic of Soriano in his church, along with Saint Francis. Another novena to Saint Cajetan was begun in the church of Our Lady of the Mercies, which ended on [the saint's] own day, and none of this placated the ire of God. Without doubt the fault was on the part of men, as the Lord has promised his mercy to anyone who values it.

Many who came down with this illness were overcome with such
a terrible frenzy (much like other plagues in the world) that they
saw strange frights and sorrows, and one morning, when the Bethlehemite fathers were in their church tending to their divine offices,
one of the sick in the room was overcome and, naked as he found
himself, jumped out of bed, went out to the cloisters, climbed up to
a very high one, and through a tiny window he threw himself to
the street below, head first. Others attempted with frightening fury
to tear apart all those present, and others executed various foolish
acts. By all paths there was nothing but the experience of sorrows,
as among the Indian dwellings and cemeteries, it was the dogs that
buried human bodies in their entrails.

The poison of the disease and its contagion were such that, in
lying on the clothing and trappings of those who had died, dogs
caught it and died on the spot. Even the donkeys that served in the
houses as carriers were killed by simply smelling the beds of the
caretakers who took them out to the stables. All the circumstances
were frightening in this tribulation, as many, in the desperation into
which they fell, uttered temerities and did scandalous things, and
they died thus.

A mestiza, whom the disease caught pregnant, gave birth without
difficulty, but, as she found herself alone (as everyone was in a general confusion), she took the placenta there beside her, having ejected
it from her entrails, and, devouring it by the mouthful, at that point
she died, followed by her newborn son. A great number of women
died in childbed, and at the same time their children, such that wher-
ever one turned one's eyes one encountered so many tears that there
are not sufficient words to describe.

It was also a notable thing to see those miserable Indians, who had
been so doggedly treated by Spaniards and Blacks (as these latter, as
slave dogs are wont to do, would steal their hats and ponchos as they
passed through the streets, obliging them to clean the filth and cor-
rals, causing them, these and others, many vexations with unspeak-
able shame), from these God took their lives and carried them away
to rest in glory, and here there remained those who had mistreated
them to experience intolerable labor and lack of everything, because
(as I have already said) without Indians this republic was left like a
body without hands or feet.

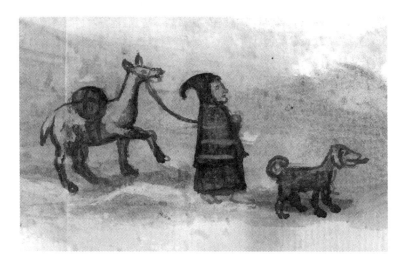

FIG. 7. An Indigenous woman with a dog and pack llama, near La Plata, circa 1639. Courtesy of Lilly Library, Indiana University, Bloomington.

Saturday, August 12, there began another novena in the main church for the new brotherhood of Saint Michael to this glorious archangel as its patron, to Saint John the Baptist in the image of his beheading, and to Saint Mary Magdalene, which ended with the sermon preached by the very reverend father Fray Juan de Relúz, of the Seraphic order, and with a very devout procession accompanied by the whole villa.

On August 14 they buried Juan Fernández, noble son of this villa, eighty years old, who always lived with the fear of God and exemplary virtues. He died on Friday, August 11, at the hour when our Redeemer was placed on the cross [on Good Friday], and since he was poor he was carried to the chapel of Our Lady of the Misericordia, and, at the same hour on the fourth day, he was buried in the church of the Misericordia. There accompanied his body, aside from the confraternity, [Potosí's] clergy, town council, nobility, and folk. Two hours before his burial, at the request of both estates, ecclesiastical and secular, three public scribes and two special ones gave faithful testimony: [they were] Francisco Jiménez and Juan de Zúñiga, plus Francisco Gutiérrez of the town council, and finally the two [select] notaries, one of the Inquisition and one ordinary, of how four full days had passed since [Juan Fernández] died of that fearsome epidemic, when the bodies of others who died were so corrupt within two hours of death that their houses could not be occupied, the body of Juan Fernández was quite tractable, incorrupt and of a most gentle and extraordinary scent, as they moved it from one side to another, and it seemed to be alive and an agreeable expression was on his venerable face. The [corregidor] general don Manuel de Villavicencio and the aldermen carried the body, which was placed in an urn and buried.

Before the burial the very reverend father Fray Gaspar de Mariaca, most dignified *comendador* of the Mercedarians, prelate of very amiable traits and virtues, knowing the good life of Juan Fernández and the circumstances of his death, he pleaded most earnestly that they give him that body, that it might be buried with the decency required by someone who had served the Lord his whole life. But the confraternity of the Misericordia did not wish it, saying that God had sent them that one, his servant. For many years Juan Fernández had dressed in the habit of the Third Order of Saint Francis. He usually took sacraments in the Jesuit church, and, from six in the morning until masses finished, he did not move from that church, and he was much given over to prayers and mortifications. The commotion of the folk amid the precious death of the just has always been observed as sure testimony of their saintliness and a convincing argument of their glory. That which occurred with the death of Juan Fernández in this villa was most notable.

[On] August 15, the day of Our Lady of the Assumption, is in this villa the feast day of the Misericordia, as it is done in that church, and it was most memorable due to the fear with which all of us awaited the eclipse of the sun, of which we had been warned by the cosmographer Dr. don Pedro de Peralta Barnuevo y Rocha, professor of mathematics of the University of San Marcos in Lima.[12] It began at eleven in the morning and lasted under an hour, and with its effects the epidemic and plague squeezed harder, and on that day alone 120 people died. With the just fear of its effects, many made general confessions, and the timorous confessed and took communion, tucked inside the churches, awaiting the will of God.

12. Presumably, the warning came from the 1719 edition of Peralta Barnuevo's almanac, *El conocimiento de los tiempos*.

The plague continued with greater force after this eclipse, and there occurred a terrible shortage of everything, and in the royal mint alone there died 130 workers, and they had to shut down, as there was no one who knew how to cut the silver [coin blanks], nor other tasks. The greater part of the Ribera [silver-refinery sector] stopped functioning, as the mita Indians all perished, and the only ones left working were paid wages, and these double. Of the famous pickmen of the Cerro, born and raised in this villa, 140 died, leaving a great void. In the slaughterhouse for small livestock, there died 40 Indians, such that no one was left to butcher at a time when meat was most needed. Of the oven keepers and other bakery workers, there died 300 people, which was enough to stop all this work. Among the tradesmen the loss and shortage was lamentable, as only 4 phlebotomists remained, there having died 38, and there was no one left to give one a bleeding, such that folks did this for one another. Of shoemakers, 46 died; tailors, 72; carpenters, 39; and thus with the rest, altogether leaving a very great need.

The circumstances of this disaster were such that one saw how God had withheld the punishment of sins so as to discharge it on this occasion in many ways, as many daughters who disobeyed and ignored the desires of their parents got married a year or two before, they died in childbed and their children with them. Many sons who did the same died speedily, leaving their female companions widowed, those who had so disgusted their parents. Others who stole to maintain their lusts died sorrowfully next to their female lovers, and they the same, alongside their male lovers, because, as everything was confusion, there were no priests nor good people to separate them, and not only this but, as they perished, they left their babies alone in that miserable state.

It was already the end of August when the maestro don Carlos Gambarte y Quiroga, grandson of the field marshal Antonio López de Quiroga (of whom and of whose great wealth in this villa we have spoken in other parts of this *History*) was received as priest of the parish of Saint Martin upon the death of the schoolmaster don José de Escarza, who died of the contagion.[13] Being so noble, charitable, and full of virtues; seeing that there were so many poor Spaniards and mestizos dead that there was now no room in two churches and

---

13. See also Bakewell, *Silver and Entrepreneurship.*

the cemetery, [Gambarte] pled kindly that they be carried to [the church of] Saint Martin, as it had much capacity in four extended corners of its cemetery. He was obeyed, and it was a great good, and there they took them, which each day were twelve, fourteen, or sixteen [cadavers], and this pious curate buried them personally with double solemnity, music, and tolls [from church bells], and, when [he was] tired, he was helped by two other priests.

And with this the confraternity of La Misericordia was assisted, as there was no longer any strength nor anyone to help them to bring out each day from the houses each one of the dead, and thus to such a distant barrio as San Martín each sufferer carried his dead one (as the plague had already lasted six months), and with this there was less sorrow in the main plaza, where, by order of the priests of the main church, the brotherhood placed them in the chapels while burying many bodies for pay. The same diligence was done with the expired Indians, carrying [their corpses] from their houses to the parish of Saint Roch.

Honors and praise are like clothing, as the most precious are not the best ones but rather the best fitted. The richest outfit, if not cut to measure for the one who displays it, serves not to brighten but rather to slight. This most benign priest of San Martín has other traits worthy of celebration, but his charity on this and all other occasions fit him very well.

Beginning in the month of August, it was introduced in this villa, also so that Most Holy Mary might intercede for it in this destruction, that they sing the holy rosary in the streets, going out from Santo Domingo on all the feast days and on Sundays each week, except Tuesday and Saturday, when, according to custom, it is sung at night. It is sung to the sound of two harps and other instruments, which is a glory on earth and without doubt must really please the Lord.

The alderman don Juan de Otálora, upon seeing the eagerness and poverty of certain poor who carried their dead to [the parish church of] San Martín but could not ask that the sepulchers be opened, for lack of means, at his own cost and at the expense of some of his fellow councilors (although this aid was not permanent), they opened up a deep ossuary at the back of the church's side chapel and another on the narrow side, which is the one that helped (but the big one was very costly, as it was a rocky site) so that they might bury with

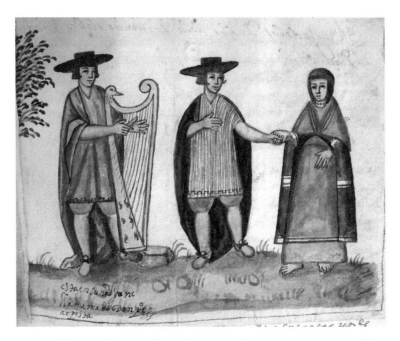

FIG. 8. Indigenous harpist and couple, near La Plata, circa 1639. Ramírez del Águila, *Noticias políticas de Indias*. Courtesy of Lilly Library, Indiana University, Bloomington.

greater ease. And putting layers of quicklime on the bodies placed side by side, and another layer of dirt on top, it thus went climbing [i.e., filling up with cadavers].

And, with this good work, they alleviated [suffering], and their charity remained and shall remain renowned, as every day he [Otálora] personally attended with his brothers, bringing the Indians from the work of his refinery to put the bodies in the ossuary and cover them with lime and earth, such that if it were not thus his charity would be incomplete. This [trait] was very strong in this gentleman, and, being generous as he was, aided by the favorable wind of divine grace, he gave full sail to love of his homeland, crossing immense seas of difficulty. And without his charity being frightened, nor avoiding untested routes, nor [diverted by] the fatal image of many dangers (as are gossip and the fear of destitution for oneself and others), he went swiftly to carry out such a heroic enterprise. May God repay him in this life and in the next.

From about the middle of August, there began to enter this afflicted villa the new crop of draftees for the annual mita, who, seeing the death toll, these Indians went to bed that night but disappeared the next morning from their dwellings, returning to their provinces and pueblos, four by four and ten by ten, leaving everything to their headmen, including their livestock and victuals, these leaders being left to suffer the displeasure of the refinery owners, but neither these nor anyone else could do anything other than lament deeply the sad state of this villa. There also perished many Indians who could not get away, and this was the inheritance left them by the dead.

The greatest and most incomparable sorrow that in this desolation broke pained hearts was [seeing] the more than eight hundred babies at the breast who remained without mothers, they and the pious women who wandered from house to house with them, looking for others who were breastfeeding and might have milk to feed them. Oh, what pain, for, having carried one of them myself with my own hands (as her mother, already sick from the contagion, expired) to a certain noble and pious lady, whereupon I found that she was already with four other babies, two little Spanish girls and the other two, little Indian girls, giving them one by one her pious breasts. I was struck dumb to see her thus, but the tears in my eyes spoke, and her piety understanding me, she asked for this fifth infant and gave it her breasts, and, although knowing that she was the daughter of noble yet poor parents (the father first succumbing to the same illness), she kept her [i.e., this orphan child] and is still raising her. There were no wet nurses, as all had perished, and, if they managed to get well, they had absolutely no milk. A multitude of orphans remained, aged one to twelve, and the luckier ones were those that died with their parents, which were many.

One saw nothing in the streets but funeral clothes, now absent the cochineal [red] capes and Spanish blues, which a few of [whose wearers] were "equalized," and the same was seen in certain Peruvians [i.e., locally born elites], because (as always) divine justice comes mixed with mercy. But among the women generally they were seen in the churches, streets, plazas, and houses in mourning veils, because all of them were touched by a smaller or greater part of the pain, and thus this villa [of Potosí] lost its luster, having always expended so much on profane things.

Spring came near (which in our hemisphere begins on September 23), and the star of Mars began to lose some of the fire of its color, and the same occurred with its effects, as the number of deaths began to diminish, no longer being eighty, sixty, or fifty per day but rather thirty or forty, and, although at the time the number of sick was over twelve thousand, the larger portion began to escape with God's mercy and intercession of she who is the Mother of sinners and by that of the saints to whom so many pleas had been made.

The annual performance of the apologies [*desagravios*] of Christ our Lord [Exaltation of the Holy Cross?] that usually begins sometime in September (as has been said in its place) was suspended this year, with great sadness among those of us who remained alive, as it was the right time. It was decided not to celebrate this year for two reasons: first, because the Jesuit fathers were attending at all hours to confessing the sick and could not stop doing so; second, because, with the heat inside the church (from such crowds), some of the convalescents who would by necessity have attended could have communicated the contagion to those who remained healthy. The town council and the fathers agreed to suspend [the gathering], and thus they canceled it.

On Tuesday, September 19, in the same week as the suspended function of the apologies, for the consolation of this villa, there began in the parish of Saint Martin a supplicatory novena to the miraculous image of Our Lady of Purification, or Candlemas, which the whole town attended since the plague had not ceased, and on Wednesday, twenty-seventh of this month, they performed a procession in which this lady went out, along with Saint Martin and Saint Roch, accompanied by everyone in town who remained healthy. Another most devout novena was done in the [monastery of] La Merced to Our Lady of Solitude, [patron] of the merchants, whose refuge was sought by all the residents of this villa. The weather was in revolt, which commonly happens in times of plague, and here it seemed that winter [*sic*] came on instead of spring, in that it did not freeze as is normal but rather it was terribly hot.

Strange occurrences did not fail to continue, as there was an Indian headman (of a certain parish in this villa) who was married but committed adultery with a young Indian woman from another parish, and it was impossible to pry him away from her. Her relatives, seeing that by no other means could they divert his feelings, convened with the adulterer to sign a writ of separation, with a cash fine plus several pounds of wax for the Lord should he return to that torrid affair. On the second day after doing this, he went back to her, taking her hands, and, as he started to break her down again, he fell dead, and, although he had not been touched by the plague, his body was instantly corrupted and [marked] with the same signs as if he had died of the sickness.

One of the town bullies, who strutted around threatening lives with words and deeds, such a sure-shot rock thrower that he never missed a head, standing one day with others of his sort, he said he did not fear death and that when it came he would face it standing, and he would wrestle it head-on. Without even finishing what he was saying, [the bully] was shoved up against a window by some [unseen] thing, and, calling for the hand of his female friend (who happened to be there) to hang onto, he was struck dead, smashed [against the window frame] but not thrown out, as he had said [i.e., meeting death standing]. Of the most famous ones of this ilk, thieves and expert stone throwers, many of them murderers not punished by human justice, were punished by the divine, as the contagion carried off to another life twenty-eight of them.

Scipio Africanus said that one has more to fear from the idle than from one's enemies, because the latter are already known. Sloth incites evils and it is not easy to prevent its invasions. Judges should seek a remedy for this evil, for at least in this villa it has always grown to the detriment of the public good. There should not be permitted in the republic people of slothful profession without knowing how they live and sustain themselves.

Let us go forward with other occurrences that came about amid the destruction. Certain young, married Spanish men who for fun dressed up as dead people for Carnival and thus enshrouded themselves, begging alms and singing responses, died of the plague in the month of August, and in the same manner that amid their jests they prepared shrouds and the rest, thus they saw themselves on the same day buried by the alms collected in various rounds for the purpose, and in the same way that their wives cried in jest and feigned dying of sorrow, in truth they died right after their husbands.

Many of those who lived through this plague ended up (without being relatives or having any other obligation) with the goods and jewels of the dead, and they buried them at minimal cost or dropped them in [front of the church of] La Misericordia without even a burial shroud. But many of these also had their lives taken by the plague, and, as they had done to others, others treated them the same way. "The turbulent river is a boon to fishermen," says the proverb, and thus it was seen on this occasion, as by many paths came many fishermen. And, finally, amid such a terrible and generalized illness, it was only the esteemed priests serving Spaniards, Indians, and Blacks who remained well amid so many burials, and in the same way the sextons and church custodians. Let us go on.

There was a certain damsel daughter whose father sent her off to learn to play various instruments, to dance, and to acquire other graces, and it so happened that the father fell ill before the plague, and, as his life was running out, although she should have felt compunction even if she were not his daughter, this one went on entertaining herself in playing the harp, singing, and dancing, with grave scandal to all those who saw it. With her father dead, she said she would not dress in mourning since he had not left her [mourning clothes], although the mother did provide these and put them on herself.

The accursed girl lost herself after [her father's] death in nine months of scandalous sensuality, acquiring two fine outfits, pearls, and other jewels. All this got in the way of her dressing in mourning, as if the acquired dresses were blackened at such and such a cost to her soul. Nine months having passed since the death of her father, the plague caught her and took hold of her and her mother, and thus others made off with all their jewels, and, if this wayward daughter said she had no mourning clothes to wear for her father, God did not wish for her to put on her gala dresses because she had been left by the one who put them on her, perhaps by force.

The drive created by the vice of lustful habits is such that the one who wants to fall into [this vice] does so quickly, putting it into effect. Like all things that fall outside the realm of reason, if quietly considered, one would not do such things. But instead of being set aside, this [vice] is pursued with longing, and, while being enacted, the [lustful acts] bring on ill feelings. [By contrast], the works of virtue do not wear one out before being enacted. Virtue has no enemies; as the heart comes rested [to virtuous acts], they are done without fatigue. I knew and communicated with this woman when she enjoyed the serenity of her damsel-hood and she only faked virtue, and then, lustful, not even for her own amusement did she find quietude.

The mortality continued, although the number [of dead] was already much smaller each day, and they could no longer carry the bodies to the distant churches, and thus they left them at night at [the church of] Saint Francis and at the doors of other churches from whence by charity they were buried. These were of the larger bodies, whereas the smaller ones [of children] appeared every morning at dawn (especially at [the church of] Saint Augustine) four, six, or ten, and all were given pious burial.

On October 19 there began in [the monastery of] Saint Francis the novena and supplication of Saint Peter of Alcántara, and on Sunday the twenty-ninth they performed his procession, in which there went out this penitent saint after a tender sermon preached by the very reverend father "president" Fray Juan de Relúz. The month of November began yet more blessed, thanks to divine mercy, by intercession no doubt of Most Holy Mary and of many saints, to whom were made so many supplications, and thus each day no more than ten, fourteen, or sixteen died.

A very notable thing occurred on the first [of November] of All Saints, since it is the custom in this devout villa to light candles for the dead in the churches from two in the afternoon until ten at night and to order responses said (in which, as I have said in its place, in this year they gathered in the main church alone more than 1,000 pesos, each [responso] costing half a real), and, although this villa was so reduced in its number of inhabitants, this pious work exceeded all others before, as in the main church and all the churches of the [regular] orders and parishes one saw lit up thirty thousand wax candles (from a quarter [pound] up to two or three pounds, more or less) such that they did not fit into the churches nor even the cemeteries, [covering] tables, and floors, and, when it comes to the accouterments of the divine cult and devotion to the souls [of purgatory], thus, as I have said, is Potosí.

This day and the following, in commemoration of the departed, the number of dead dropped again, which seemed to have occurred due to this pious function, as in all the churches and in the charity hospital they buried only eight people. This same day there reached this villa from Buenos Aires the news of the tribulations in which our king and lord Philip V, God save him, found himself, with the alliance of the [Holy Roman] Empire, France, England, and other enemies against his monarchy, from which great evils would result, a thing felt in this villa in the extreme.[14] He who brought this news was a Basque, arriving from court with the royal pouch and a decree from His Majesty, saying that for the second time there would govern as viceroy of these kingdoms the most illustrious and most excellent lord don Fray Diego Morcillo, archbishop of La Plata, and it was a notable thing to see that this mail carrier or captain of the pouch (as they are titled in this villa) came all the way from the [royal] court for this purpose alone and in a light vessel (although it still suffered storms), quickly reaching Buenos Aires and, from there to this villa, he happily walked five hundred leagues.

The town was in an uproar at this news, doubting its certitude until this captain assured them that, being an official of the royal secretary in Madrid, he knew [for certain] that which he related, having been at the assembly of the dispatches. With this, on the second day after his arrival, before dawn, in company of the general don Manuel [Potosí's corregidor] and of the lord don Pedro Vázquez, fiscal of the royal audiencia, and of Señor Antequera (Indian legal advocate just arrived from the court to take up this post), don Francisco Astigueta and many other gentlemen departed for La Plata. And His Most Illustrious Excellency, upon receiving the decree, the royal audiencia then got a special order that at that point they receive him as viceroy of these kingdoms, and thus was it done on December 4.

And, as it is already stated in another part of this *History* in the appropriate chapter according to the order we have followed, when, although for just a few days he was received as viceroy of these kingdoms [in 1716], it is not excessive to say so once again. His Excellency granted the captain who brought the royal decree the governorship of Cochabamba, which he later sold for 12,500 pesos, and His Excellency commenced his government, preparing himself for the trip to Lima via [the province of] Los Charcas without coming to this villa, as the contagion still circulated. Thus we shall leave all this and return to following the thread of the destruction the plague wrought

14. Arzáns refers to the War of the Quadruple Alliance (August 2, 1718–February 17, 1720).

on this villa, summing up this lamentable event with the number of those who perished.

Tuesday, December 7, the alderman don Juan de Otálora, city magistrate and chief justice of this villa by absence of the [corregidor] general don Manuel, made public a decree in the style of war [i.e., with fifes, drums, salutes, etc.] that everyone celebrate the reception of His Excellency [Archbishop Morcillo] as viceroy of these kingdoms, with luminaries in the streets and plazas and large candles in the balconies and windows that night, as was done, accompanied by the peal of all the church bells, which lifted the spirits, since in nine months they heard only the death knells.

How could even the most barbaric Catholic look death in the eyes and not try to prepare for a good death? Time is always short, and labors great, but capacious and quick is the mercy of God when pled for: this villa had already experienced this on this occasion and on others. But the surer thing is to have worked it out beforehand. One of humankind's greatest blind spots is that, despite knowing how God must be satisfied by the hour of death, one instead offends he who deserves so much. Careful, then, ye living: take heed the punishment of so many deaths. To fear and love God is a secure thing, dying in whatever way one might, although God punishes in general, and it is a sorrowful tragedy, as the just and unjust, the innocent and guilty, all perish. Ten months—with the last of December of this memorable year—did God sustain the plague and epidemic, although (blessed and admired be his mercy) this month having passed, it ceased to the extent that there no longer died more than one, two, or four per day, and on one day none died, and, although there were many sick, the majority got well quickly.

I have already said how the plague caught this villa with [a population of] sixty thousand souls of all nations, statuses, sexes, and ages, the greater part being Indians, they totaling thirty-five thousand. Among these the greatest destruction was wrought, and in the end (in ten months), counted by my personal diligence, there died over twenty-two thousand of all statuses, between both sexes, large and small, within this villa, as it has no extramural [neighborhoods] nor suburbs: a notable loss and most lamentable now and for years to come.

To this one must add the destruction of the Indian villages in the near hinterland, in which there died of the same plague ten thousand people, and there were even those pueblos that lacked anyone to bring victuals to this villa or even to cultivate the fields for this purpose. The nearest villages that by truck and trade maintain this villa in victuals are twelve, and all were destroyed: Caiza, Porco, Puna, Chaqui, Tambo de Bartolo, Siporo, Chulchucani, Potobamba, Tacobamba, Tinguipaya, Salinas, and Tarapaya, not counting another twelve towns farther out that were also destroyed by the same contagion and that likewise provisioned this villa.

In the city of La Plata and its outskirts they experienced the same destruction and in the city of Oruro and its satellites, likewise, such that according to what was said it [i.e., the pandemic] ran down to the lower [Pacific coast] provinces and to Lima, and it proved an indiscriminate destruction. One may conjecture that in the three years since it reached Buenos Aires from Europe, in a space of more than six hundred leagues up to the end of this year [1719] there perished two hundred thousand persons.

And, finally, as for destructions of this villa by way of mass death, none had been like this one, for the memorable civil wars named for the Vicuñas lasted four years [1622–25], and in those there perished at the hands of men some six thousand persons, minus four thousand wounded who did not die. In the flood of the Cari Cari reservoir [of 1626] in the three hours it lasted (as already noted in its place in this *History*), there perished four thousand, but in this one and in a few brief months the number surpassed twenty-two thousand.

Thus does God punish sins. And with all the novenas and supplications; so many pleas; sermons delivered with such frequency (those of the novenas alone totaling thirty-three); so many processions displaying modesty, compunction, and Christian piety (as with the one they did on November 12 with the most beautiful and miraculous image of Our Lady of the Rosary after her annual novena, [these added up to] twenty); with so many mortifications, secret and public; with so many acts of charity done by the good; and with so many tender innocents, parish priests, most virtuous regular clergy, and "persons of the century" [like Juan Fernández], God-fearing as they died, I do not know if divine justice has been satisfied.

Potosí wails and cries for having experienced such a grave malady, and it fears only its total ruin as consequence, without seeing that all human prosperity is only a gust of wind that blows in all directions. Without scarcity there is no bonanza, yet if it grows it is a tempest.

Finally, one may consider that life is an oil lamp, glass and fire: glass made when blown with a breath, and a fire that with a breath goes out. These are, have been, and shall be, Potosí, the glories of your famed Cerro and of your memorable villa. That which has weighed most and which has shined brightest in you has been and remains your riches. And what are these riches but a trial at the start, a care for later, and a mere sentiment for the beyond? What more are they? A magnet for vice, an occasion for envy, a cause for disputes, and, what is more, a path that leads you to hell should you not use them well. . . .

[After describing a petition to the newly appointed archbishop-viceroy to end the mita labor draft, Arzáns adds the following note before ending discussion of the year 1719:] His Most Illustrious Excellency ordered this guild [of Potosí silver refiners] to whitewash the huts and other mita Indians' dwellings, as lime is an antivenin against the contagion, and thus they did, these buildings never before having been seen whitened but rather blackened by continuous smoke.

## Chapter XLIX

How the plague continued in the provinces of Charcas and Porco as in the other provinces of this kingdom, doing great damage to this villa, among other trials experienced within it.

[Arzáns begins the first chapter on the year 1720 by lamenting the general shortage of good governors, while suggesting that Potosí's corregidor during the pandemic, Gen. Manuel de Villavicencio y Granada, was above average.[15] He then returns to the plague.]

The cruel plague continued in this villa but fell off considerably at the start of this year, but in some of the surrounding provinces it maintained the same rigor, and in others it increased again, adding to the tribulations of this overwhelmed villa, as none could supply victuals and other things necessary for human life. It has already been noted in previous chapters how by careful numeration those who died [in Potosí] totaled twenty-two thousand among both sexes,

15. Arzáns may be dissimulating, as Corregidor Villavicencio was later exiled by Viceroy Morcillo; see *Libros de acuerdos*, 4:108.

all statuses, and all ages. Several more were added to this number at the beginning of this year, although with respect to what was later seen in Cuzco and other towns, what happened in this villa was merciful, and divine grace was most resplendent in that few died without receiving the holy sacraments, as has been said.

Among the several signs of this divine grace is one that (according to the books of the Third Order of our father Saint Francis, whose current rector is father Fray Alonso de Olazábal) there died, in the eleven months of [the pandemic's] duration up to February 20 of this year, 2,665 persons of this [religious] order alone, professed or having professed at the very end of their lives, minus another 300 who escaped [alive] among both sexes, and all of these dressed themselves during convalescence in the holy habit of the Third [Order of Franciscans].

His [Divine] Majesty may wish in his infinite mercy that this punishment be our lesson so that the memory of it reins us in so as not to throw ourselves into our guilt, running headlong in our vices without fear, since although the Lord punishes them, his father's love obliges him to mitigate his ire and to mix his mercy with his punishment, and it hurts him that after so many lashes we remain so asleep, and if we awaken from our lethargy it is not to mend things as we should. Potosí wept at its loss, its hinterland wailed at its ruin, and with this the Lord warned the inhabitants of the other provinces of the threat so that they would know that, as he had here discharged the lash, his arm was not too tired to do the same there should they fail to demonstrate repentance for their sins.

The rigorous plague went on spreading this year, and before the month of December started, the towns of Oruro, Cochabamba, and Tarija were already destroyed, with innumerable Indian towns, as well as La Paz, Arequipa, and Cuzco, and in this last one the destruction was greatest, as there was found an innumerable Native population, and letters from that city affirmed that in six months there died seventy thousand people, and if one were to continue to the third year, which was 1721 (to complete that which was said by the cosmographer of the city of Lima [Peralta Barnuevo], that for the three hours that the [August 15, 1719] eclipse of the sun lasted, there would correspond three years of sickness, such that this plague would be suffered in all the provinces all the way to Lima, and from there God would take it as far as he wished), and, without entertaining doubt, from Buenos Aires to Lima, it carried off more than half a million people, according to the various accounts, which would be in a space of one thousand leagues, all the way to Abancay, and by careful count and computation it surpassed four hundred thousand people.

This plague still continued through the month of February in the city of La Plata, and from there they sent to this villa a decree with the order that under penalty of excommunication that we cease or stop the running of the bulls during Carnival and in the days leading up to it, as had been done there. The decree was appealed and the ecclesiastical vicar suspended its execution, seeing that the villa and its judges had already spent the money, only wanting to entertain the town after a full year of so much suffering, as misfortunes are not remedied with spite but rather they get worse, and, what is more, this tired villa had no other entertainment than this, which was quite short at the end of this year, when (as has been written in this *History*) it has had in the past extremely lavish ones.

And it was only fair what was done with this decree since in that city [of La Plata] they had held their fiestas of Our Lady of Guadalupe, which always includes a running of free-range bulls, when Potosí was in the midst of its worst affliction ever and when the head of the confraternity [of Guadalupe] and other respectable persons asked that it be suspended. But no attention was paid to the trials of this villa; rather, they added another two days of bulls on top of the usual ones, and with these they spent six days in fiestas. But, as they were just starting to bait those bulls in that city, the plague came on slowly, and later it picked up, although with some mercy.

There are many men who go about fussing over the lives of others as their own lives run to ruin; they are the sweepers of customs. Those who sweep the streets have to scour to sweep them, and thus they leave them without dust and without mud. The streets are left clean, yet they [the sweepers] are left covered with the same dust and mud. Those who gossip about the actions of others and find fault in other republics [i.e., cities] hurt themselves and the one they target even if made of stone, but they are obliged to mend their ways: they or the republic must make amends, and [still] they carry the blemish of being foulmouthed.

The diversion of the bulls and the joy of Carnival (which this year for fear of the plague was not prejudicial to souls) having passed, and, entering into Easter and especially the start of March, they performed the annual novena of Saint Francis Xavier that began on the third, with great devotion by exhortation from the Jesuit fathers and in particular the learned father Miguel de Estrada, who asked that everything possible be done in his festival sermons (which he preached on Easter Sundays to the inhabitants of this villa), that they plead with God that by intercession of their patron Xavier that he drop from his divine hands at last the lash of the plague that was still being felt, and thus it happened since from this ten-day period onward the Lord seemed to mitigate his ire.

The lamentable and perhaps hopelessly irremediable custom in this villa of homicide did not cease, despite the experience of the terrible destruction of the plague, such that in the first four months of this year there died tragically five women at the hands of their very same male companions (out of lust), and in the same stretch of time there were killed another seven men in diverse streets and fields.

At the start of March, it was learned in this villa that the ships that left Buenos Aires the previous year loaded with silver came back from the Bank [near Buenos Aires] for having been spotted by various enemies there nearby, everyone feeling for those the delay of their desired voyage. Oh, unhappy and pitiful depths of human nature, ever ambitious for its own advancement but blind in making choices and searching for the right means to gain eternal rest.

At the beginning of the month of April, there reached this villa by ordinary post news from His Catholic Majesty Philip V, God save him, that it was determined by his Indies Council to end the mita so as to cleanse his royal conscience and to remediate the damage that maintaining it had done to the Indians, thanks to the repeated complaints of the opposite side against the illustrious guild of silver refiners, informed of the ill treatment they had meted out, when in truth there was much sinister information in those reports from the opposite side.

But as the lord protector of the Indians, Fiscal Antequera (who, as I have noted, had just arrived in this villa the previous year to take up this new post) came charged by His Majesty to enact precisely this decree and to look after the Natives, as they were free (the motive behind the order to end the mita, as his predecessor, Charles II, of glorious memory, had already mandated), for this reason the lord fiscal began to put together writings in favor of the Indians, although this resolution did not go into effect because the most illustrious and most excellent don Fray Diego Morcillo [the interim viceroy] suspended it as someone who saw the present case, even advertising the inconveniences that would invariably follow if executed and in particular the destruction of fourteen curates (not counting that of Saint Roch of El Tío) that had been erected in this villa for these Indians of the mita, which bring together seventeen provinces, and, although by cutting them in half they might not all perish, soon enough these curates would dissipate.

The document bearing this order and royal mandate had reached Lima almost two years before, addressed to the [viceroy] prince of Santo Buono, but His Excellency, considering the ills that would follow from publishing it, kept it secret, awaiting a better opportunity, and with the arrival of the lord Morcillo in Lima the two princes published it together.

Ending the mita (a matter pending for more than eighty years) is certainly holy and just, but not due to the guild of refiners (who, if the Indians serve them, they in turn sustain them and pay their travel costs) but rather because of another two parties that gain from the mita, which are its captains [i.e., recruiters] and the lord priests, whose judgment must be left only to God, who sees the good and the bad.

This royal decree on this particular said not only to end the [mita] of Potosí but also that of [the mercury-mining town of] Huancavelica, although this pertained only to that royal audiencia [of Lima] for its mercury, a substance also ordered sent out from Spain to New Spain (but this one for Peru has very great difficulties [referring to the mines of Almadén in La Mancha versus Huancavelica]) and that, in exchange for denying the mita to the silver refiners of this Imperial Villa, the royal fifth [silver tax] would be reduced to a tenth. In another clause His Majesty promised to take over the role played by the silver merchants and pay the [mill owners] directly at nine pesos per mark [of raw silver] rather than at six and a half pesos, as is standard in this villa, but none of this was put into practice.

Of the last cases having to do with this plague, as strange as they were exemplary (to which we continue referring), there were seen in this villa, for punishment of its sins, one among certain obstinate sinners who in plain view of the destruction did not stop offending God. A certain married man, an outsider, committed adultery with a lost and very scandalous woman, of the sort so esteemed by foolish men, and for this he developed such abhorrence for his proper wife (despite being noble, quite young, and very beautiful) that out of the blue one day, tearing her flesh with most cruel lashes and other mistreatments, he had her locked up in a convent of nuns, where she was kept two months, denied all food.

It so happened that, after fifty-six days of this mistreatment had passed, these adulterers being asleep one night, the [adulterous] woman was awakened by frightening voices saying that some fearsome Blacks would whip her to pieces, and, her adulterous lover being unable to detain her, she leaped out of bed and, while trying to open the door to the parlor, she fell dead. The adulterous man shouted to his servants, so filled with fear he could barely articulate words, and all gathering together they found the adulterous woman with a frightening expression on her face, and her whole body appeared to have been whipped with burning rods, such that they did not even dare to pull the body away from the door, and, going to another room, where an aunt of this woman stayed, she serving as procuress in those ridiculous affairs, they also found her dead with signs of the plague, which she had contracted only one day earlier.

This occurred in the month of April of this year [of 1720], and, although they tried to keep it entirely secret, eventually one of the servants declared it to a priest, who right away asked me to write about it as an example for adulterers and that, if God permits the innocent to suffer, it is so that he might punish the guilty with greater rigor. After the death of this adulteress, they found in one of her desks two wax forms, dressed, one with her clothing and of the same fabric she wore and the other of the man, united by the arms, and a tiny piece of magnetic stone pressed into the form of the woman, along with other filthy details, all of which they threw into an arroyo.

The male adulterer with that fearsome event opened his eyes from blindness, went afterward to the convent, called on his wife, begged her pardon, and took her home, where they now live very properly and the husband in repentance of all. Of the adulteress God only knows what happened, as her life was most dissolute and without fear of the divine, entertained by lusts, carried along by such an evil path that is witchcraft, the means by which the devil induces lost women so as to entrap them without alerting them that the determined will to sin at all hours makes the hour of death most dangerous and that long custom takes on the stubborn determination of nature.

On top of so much calamity suffered by this villa, there grew as well the inability to alleviate its poverty, because the chunks of silver they took from the Cerro [Rico], even as they were few, the greater part were carried off by men from Spain to the port of Arica, to Ilo [Peru], and elsewhere, where once again there were found French ships with clothing, of which in the months of April and May they introduced large quantities into this villa secretly, the richest merchants lending a hand to this effect, as the ordinary desire of the ambitious is that there be many who do it, as it is in all evil things, either to have less than they claim or for having more with which to excuse oneself. It's a miracle if not everyone follows that which many do. With this it would not be found very strange that this or that person does the same.

The disgraces caused by the custom of homicide carried on even among the men of greater account and credit, such that in the month of April, one Saturday night, over matters of honor Lorenzo de los Ríos, a Biscayner, who went accompanied by a certain Juan Antonio, a Galician youth, killed Lorenzo de Navedas, a son of this villa, and all three of them merchants. The killer escaped from the hands of the judge, and there it ended with him losing only his credit and estate. This was not the only disgrace that happened among Spaniards, as on Saturday, May 25, José de Mendivera, a youth of quite harmful customs, living in the house of Blas de Castro, an old man of good lifestyle who sustained that fierce killer and even shared his capital with him, [the youth] blinded by greed and instigated by the devil, seeing [the old man] ill and incapacitated, he set about trying to strangle him, and, not being able to abbreviate his life, he took a pair of scissors out of his pocket and gave him a cruel wound on the nape of his neck, from which he later died without sacraments nor any disposition of his capital, from which that perverse man stole all he could, and, when he saw that that justice officers found out, he retired to a monastery, and there he remained without the least punishment.

The unfortunate Blas de Castro should well have feared the evil that befell him, as he knew some of the perverse customs of his murderer, but he was not quite persuaded that there could be a friend so infamous as to harm the one who sustains him, but it's not the first time in the world that this has happened, and, if human intelligence knew how to govern the future, it would rob the stars of this exercise, weakening their influences and annulling destinies. To predict evils is not to avoid them. To be good or bad is in one's own hands, to be lucky or to be cursed, in the judgments of heaven. The most that prudence can do to better divine [i.e., predict] is to temper the evils with precautions. What one can always do is prepare the soul to suffer them.

No fewer sorrows were experienced similarly in the remaining months of this year, as on the day of July 27, when, bringing the body of a girl of thirteen or fourteen to the chapel of Our Lady of the Misericordia to bury her in the main church, noticing that the shroud that enveloped her from head to toe was tightly sewn, such that very little of the face could be seen, they opened it up to see her neck and shoulders to find that she had been cut up and killed by extremely cruel blows, as they soon found all over the cadaver. They alerted justice officers, and they found out that she had been cut up by a certain mestiza and two men, and this woman was jailed, but the whole thing led nowhere. Ten more luckless ones were killed at the hands of their enemies up to the end of this year, and they counted more than thirty badly injured, and all of these evil deeds were driven by lust.

How many people in this world would be fortunate if only they knew to avoid the most cruel knock of this passion, and by not avoiding it they give their bodies over to dishonor, their souls over to sin, their reputations over to infamy, their capital sacked, and their lives to an infinity of inquietudes and torments, and many times to lose their life, body, and soul? Oh terrible passion! Oh lust! And in what subjection you hold the world! For you they bribe and steal away the most respectable damsels; they destroy families; the ungrateful sons bring about the deaths of their parents. It is because of you that there are so many young widows in the world suffering dishonor; so many of this feminine sex who, after having falsely served in the big cities, die in a poor hospital; so many innocent dead by a death that precedes even their birth; so many children thrown out into the world like froth from the sea, handed off to poverty and vice. It is because of you, oh insatiable passion, disturbing and upsetting even the most chaste marriages. For you they use poison and the cord [to strangle], swords are sharpened, and tragedies begin in the shadows of the night, only to end on a scaffold in the middle of the day. All these evils are brought about by lust.

Although in the previous year it seemed that Potosí had already been totally destroyed with the great mortality, as has already been

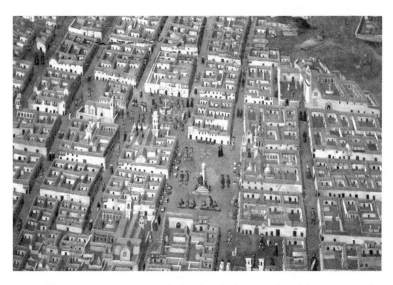

FIG. 9. The Potosí city center with the chapel of Our Lady of the Misericordia church (now gone) at the upper end of the main square, upper left (number 11). Detail from Gaspar Miguel de Berrío's *The Imperial City and Rich Hill of Potosí*, circa 1758. Courtesy of Museo Colonial de Charcas, Sucre, Bolivia. Photo by the author.

said, and that from there on one would see its "imperial" town site deserted, but it did not happen thus, as in this [year] it filled back up with folks of all types, such that it surpassed the number of fifty-six thousand persons, and each day there came in from the various provinces more and more to settle permanently, and thus they celebrated the feasts of the divine cult with great pomp, such that the processions of Holy Week exceeded those of other years, and in those of Corpus [Christi] huge and extraordinary altars were constructed, some of them covered on top with damask-wrapped candles, it having been many years since this had been done due to the obstacles involved, and in particular those who made it happen were Juan Camacho de Pila and Andrés Pontejos, merchants, helping out with the money that each one had got pledged from other persons in the business community.

These two devout merchants had their altar assembled in the little plaza next to the cemetery of the church of Our Lady of La Merced, the site given by the reverend father *comendador* to Andrés Pontejos

with total freedom, as he was one of the majordomos of [the confraternity of] Our Lady of Solitude, founded by the businesspeople
of this villa in that church. He had put together at great cost and
with remarkable diligence a triangular altar in the Tuscan order with
three arches and as many facades, having closed off the opening to
the street with planks to the height of six statures [ca. thirty-three
feet]. The arch in the middle (more elevated than the collateral ones)
and its highest cupula were covered with beautiful mirrors with
gilded frames and artificial foliage and in the same way the collateral
cupulas. The frontispiece, crowns, and cornices were covered in the
same manner with crystalline mirrors, garnished with foliage on rich
silks. In the place of the pedestals up to the bench and its overhang,
they placed three gilded and very spacious octagonal stairs, which
they covered with mirrors in gilded frames and pictures of admirable
design.

Upon these three steps were many cherubs dressed in gold and
silver, and their heads adorned with bright and colorful feathers,
fastened with ivy and laurel in the savage fashion, flowerpots, and
bouquets, with other curiosities and finery, such that it all caused
much happiness. The frontals, wire mesh, and candlesticks were all of
the very finest silver. On the tops of the steps that faded into pyr-
amids were seen the finest writing desks, inlaid with tortoise shell,
ebony, and ivory, garnished with silver, and in all the corridors and
cornices they placed more "savage" cherubs with the same outfits as
those aforementioned. Three arches of silver of first-rate craftsman-
ship stood in the eminences of each of these triangles, and in the middle, below the principal cupula, there was a gilded tabernacle with a
crystalline mirror of extraordinary size, and there the monstrance of
the Lord, on the right-hand side an image of the lord [King] Philip V,
God save him (with rich clothing and jewels of the most precious
stones, with a sword in the right hand, with the left taking the baton
as if defending the faith), and on the left side the Turk as opponent
(also adorned with jewels and precious stones, such that in the images
of these two princes were seen more than 100,000 pesos' worth of
jewels).

The entire street from one side to the other and from the tiled
roof to the ground was covered with paintings on canvas of various
histories, of Flemish and Roman scenes, of which this villa has many,
and various images of our Lord, of his Most Holy Mother, and of

the saints of the celestial court so admirably painted, and with many rich tapestries. The battlements of the cemetery were adorned in the same manner, placing in a prominent spot and beneath the canopy a portrait on canvas of the lord Philip V, and there as well [was laid out in diorama] the history of the birth of Christ our Savior in small figures, with a variety of the stages of his most holy life, and on all sides many mirrors, of which for the whole altar there totaled over 320 among large, medium, and small ones. The richness and curiosity that went beyond what has already been stated with regard to this altar was such that to write about it all would require still more belabored chapters.

The altar of the Bethlehemite hospital was also very well done, the same that they built beneath a triumphal arch in the Doric order with a Corinthian part, and the columns Solomonic, all the cornices, crowns, capitals, and pedestals garnished with mirrors, gilt frames, beautiful paintings, artificial foliage, and great curiosity and adornment. The feast and novena of Our Lady of the Rosary was also most extraordinary this year, in which the majordomo don Juan de Sante-lices, a striking "mountaineer" [*montañés*], and the other confraternity majordomos displayed the rest with care and devotion, mostly in the extremely costly adornment of the retable, the mirrors, the gilt frames, silver mesh, foliage and other innumerable curiosities, such that in all the cornices of the body of the church, altars, and facades they placed many cherubs with so much jewelry and precious stones that it was all appraised at more than 400,000 pesos. And so it was with all the other festivals so that in a certain way Potosí paid for the mercy that God showed in not totally finishing off his Imperial Villa for its sins.

At the beginning of June, the royal treasure [to be sent to Spain] amounted to 641,000 pesos in all, exceeding by a wide margin the previous year's, due to the destruction caused by the plague. The account was closed by the lord fiscal don Pedro Vázquez, as in the previous year. Of this whole amount very little remained in promissory notes, such that what was owed in silver was handed over by order to the lord don Matías de Astoraica, royal treasury official and accountant, a Peruvian from Callao, who arrived the previous year as one of three ministers of the royal treasury, most zealous and a very loyal servant of His Majesty in this charge. Of royal fifths touching on the silver refineries, there were entered 60,000 pesos less than in the year before, a most serious thing, but it was because of the lack of Indians that had occurred, such that they stopped milling [silver ore] along the main millstream.

Thursday at two in the afternoon, August 1, certain citizens announced that don Juan José de Eraso, of the Navarrese nation, a former alderman of the town council of this villa who had donated his [purchased and inheritable] post to His Majesty many years before his death, had not opened the doors of his house in eight days. They reported it to a justice officer since he did not respond when they called out, and only a mean dog that he kept growled, albeit weakly. The [corregidor] general don Manuel came and ordered the locks broken and enter[ed] with other men; the loyal brute [the dog], all but falling down from hunger (although he was most fierce), went and hid himself between the legs of his master, who was seated on a chair, quite dead and putrefied, his head placed on his hand, his hat soaked, as not even this had fallen.

They removed the corpse, and, as it was insufferable, right away the aldermen joined together to carry out his burial in the main church, and they had to put him in the sepulcher even before the sung vigil was finished, as it appeared his abdomen was about to explode.[16] It was quite a notable thing, the story of this man, who after being widowed he never wanted to take part in society, not even with a single servant, and, as with everything, one dies as one lives, and thus he died, having enjoyed the great wealth that he inherited from his wife, who herself was a rich widow, and she at sixty years of age already had married this alderman and lived another ten or twelve years before dying and leaving him as the sole heir of all she owned. Don José left nothing of much value, although in old suits of clothes and other junk he had plenty to cover the burial and so much for the judge. All that was precious he sold during his life, and, if he had silver, there was hardly anyone who did not have some of it. An example for many, this judge, who for his avarice admitted no society whatsoever.

16. Eraso's burial caused a ruckus among Potosí's churchmen. See the city council minutes in Inch, *Libros de acuerdos*, 4:96 (entry for August 1, 1720). The council seems to have barely met in the plague year of 1719.

# 2

Catastrophe in Cuzco

*Not long after Bartolomé Arzáns de Orsúa y Vela died while writing his great chronicle of Potosí in 1736, another Creole author, the priest Diego de Esquivel y Navia (ca. 1700–1779), composed a similar annalistic history of his hometown of Cuzco. Esquivel's Chronological News of the Great City of Cuzco is not as voluminous as Arzáns's History of the Imperial Villa of Potosí, but they have a similar, sermonizing flavor. For both authors the 1719–20 pandemic was a one-of-a-kind event, visible proof of God's displeasure.*

*Esquivel came from one of Cuzco's richest and most illustrious families, and he had more formal education than Arzáns, reflected in a fondness for Latin quotes. Esquivel's history starts with the Incas and goes up to the year 1749, again not unlike Arzáns's long chronicle of Potosí. Esquivel's narrative invites comparisons—for example, what did he believe caused the Cuzco outbreak? Was it preceded by portents? Who did he say was hit hardest? How long did it last, and how were victims treated? Who gets praised and who is blamed?*

*Esquivel's narrative of the year 1720 starts without the signs and wonders favored by Arzáns, but he notes that the inevitable Archbishop-Viceroy Diego Morcillo passed through Cuzco for a week or so of feasting and bullfights on his way to Lima in late December 1719 and early January 1720. Esquivel withholds judgment, but it seems the archbishop-viceroy's visit cost the city dearly in subsequent months. Esquivel adds that the English privateer John Clipperton evaded capture while raiding in the Pacific, having abducted a high-ranking Spanish couple. It is a hint if not a harbinger. Esquivel then turns to the great pestilence.*

## Chapter XXXIV

It was in the month of April 1720 that this city experienced a general epidemic fever, which began in Buenos Aires at the start of the year 1719 [*sic*] and ran through all these provinces, even beyond Guamanga [present-day Ayacucho], and by way of letters from Cádiz it was found that the Moors along the coast of Morocco had suffered from it at the same time [a potential reference to the plague that hit Marseille]. And since this plague preceded the [solar] eclipse of August 15, 1719, this could not have been one of its effects. Yet how might one properly describe the lamentable destruction we witnessed in Cuzco and the southern provinces? There are not enough voices to ponder the calamity, and too many tears would have to be shed to mourn it.

It was similar to the most memorable [plagues] we read about in histories, so violent, lethal, and voracious that it admitted no relief, nor did any medicine match it. The specific morbidity or condition was like typhus, with an intense fever and ardent body aches. This was of the abdomen and head, but the symptoms were so distinct and even contrary that one could not form a clear diagnosis, and thus a cure was rendered impossible. For some it caused frenzy and in others a bloody vomit, always fatal. Phlebotomy alleviated some and sped the departure of others, or most. Among pregnant women it was rare if one escaped. Some who overcame the fever died of dysentery. They tried out various unusual medicines and new experiments, and, as the poet said,

> War was waged on [the evil disease] with the healing arts,
> But the destruction exceeded our resources, which once con-
> quered lay in ruins.[1]

It was such that he who felt struck by this disease could not hang on to any more time in his suffering than that of his last breath, which was also said by Aeacus, *apud* Ovid, book 7 of the *Metamorphoses*:

---

1. Ovid, *Metamorphoses* 7.526–27: "Pugnatum est arte medendi / Exitium superabat opem quae victa jacebat." On Esquivel's selections translator Michael Brumbaugh notes, "This author mines quotations primarily from two passages. Ovid and Seneca were widely read during the early modern period, so these are not "deep cuts" as it were. Moreover, the author does not seem to care much about the context from which he draws his quotations. For instance, he snatches one description of plague-induced calamity right out of the middle of a sentence where it was merely a precursor to a description of societal breakdown and crime outbursts that result from plague (the main concern of the original passage)."

And hope of deliverance
Has vanished and they see an end to their disease in burial.[2]

The humor that prevailed in the human body, providing material to the infection of the pestilential and corrupt air, was constant, as certified by the physicians as being that of the choler, as is true in most epidemics. And they were persuaded, outside the common symptoms, that the headache and blood from the mouth and the black issue from the nostrils were caused by the corruption and abduction of the humors, as happened in the plague of Thebes, about which sang the [Theban] chorus (Seneca, *Oedipus*):

> Then a fiery vapor
> Burns the very stronghold of the body [i.e., the head].[3]

And further afterward:

> From the aquiline nose drips black
> blood and it bursts the gaping veins.[4]

The morbid contagion was so quick and violent that some died as soon as they received it, as seen with the barber-surgeons and others who immediately attended to the sick or who buried the cadavers. And even in this regard this plague was similar to that suffered by the people of Aegina, in which, according to the same Ovid:

> The closer someone is to a sick person and the more faithfully
> he attends him,
> The more swiftly he comes to his own death.[5]

2. Ovid, *Metamorphoses* 7.564–65: "Atque salutis / Spes abiit finemque vident funere morbi."
3. Seneca, *Oedipus* 184–85 (Chorus of Thebans to Oedipus): "tum vapor ipsam / corporis arcem flammens urit."
4. Seneca, *Oedipus* 189–90 (Chorus of Thebans to Oedipus): "Stillatque niger naris aduncae / cruor, et venas, rumpit hiantes." Michael Brumbaugh adds, "The description of the nose is probably meant to show a stark contrast between the 'perfect' nose and the devastating illness."
5. Ovid, *Metamorphoses* 7.563–64: "Quo propior quisque est, servitque fidelius ægro / In partem leti citius venit."

The surprising thing was that even the donkeys and llamas, which are the sheep of this land, on which were transported the bodies for burial in their towns and churches, most perished, emitting blood from the mouth. Such was the force of this shock, this malignant repercussion.

The city [of Cuzco] had found itself threatened since the previous year, as the news had arrived of the mortality in parts south, and, seeing that many people were in danger and that the plague was about to hit, the town council, chief justice, and officers, by way of their procurator general and two deputies, pled with the lord bishop on April 26, along with the dean and ecclesiastical assembly, prelate, regular and secular clergy, that they perform supplications and public processions in order to placate the Lord, whose lash we already had in view.

But these were not so effective, as he let loose the blow that was feared, as with each day the malady went on spreading, and there multiplied the sick and the frequency of funerals, continuous laments, and repeated tolls. As those of the church bells caused a fatal anguish, exacerbating the suffering, the bishop prohibited them, and likewise the fasts and abstinences from meat for this year and the next, such that nature might have the vigor to resist such a powerful enemy. But this [enemy] triumphed more and more each day, and, as the sun entered the sign of Leo, it displayed itself so bloody and cruel, armed with its scythe, in company of the Eumenides sisters [i.e., the Furies], captained by the inflexible and steely Atropos, that there fell in the space of a bimester many thousands.

The destruction was such that nothing like it had been seen in Cuzco since the plague of the year 1589, and yet this one was even greater than that one both in duration (from the March equinox until the month of November) and also in that in this one there died those of all ages, sexes, and stations.

No part [of society] is immune and free from destruction
But every age and sex fall to ruin alike.
Young men with old, fathers with sons,
The deadly plague yokes them together.[6]

---

6. Seneca, *Oedipus* 52–54 (from Oedipus's opening monologue): "Nec ulla pars immunis exitio vacat / Sed omni actas pariter, et sexus ruit / Juvenesque senibus jungit / et gnatis patres. Funesta pectis."

But those most bloodied by it were the miserable Indians due to their hot constitution, [the pandemic] desolating their houses, parishes, and pueblos. The least number of dead per day in the city was one hundred, and the peaks were August 6, 10, and 15, plus September 2, and of these it was on August 10 that the [daily] number surpassed seven hundred. Whatever direction one cast one's gaze, one saw nothing but dead bodies, each new day displaying the ravages done by night. At dawn the church cemeteries were found filled with bodies. "I have seen corpses abandoned in front to temple doors."[7] It is more true here.

There was no longer any space in the churches for burials, and thus they opened great trenches with much quicklime in the cathedral cemetery. And yet these also filled with the multitude of bodies such that, having nowhere to bury them, the lord bishop designated and blessed two extramural cemeteries, the first on August 12 in the site called Conchopata, south of the city, and the other a little later in Ayaguayco toward the west, and they gathered up and transported all the cadavers there from the churches, streets, and plazas in a great carriage, built especially for this purpose and paid for by a devout person.

The venerable dean and council of the cathedral ordered on August 27 that no more graves be opened inside the churches. And in such confusion in which no one observed funeral rites anymore for lack of time and ministers, and all the people prostrate, it came about that one saw many bodies eaten by dogs for lack of anyone to collect them. Consumed as they were with such a voracious appetite, these animals, after having enjoyed for the first time the taste of human flesh, they traveled in packs to snatch the meager spoils, reaching the point of threatening the living, who could extinguish their brazenness only with firearms and other weapons.

In the provinces of Collao [near Lake Titicaca], the plague was so astronomical that they were nearly left deserted, dying each day twenty, thirty, or forty, more or less, depending on the size of the towns. Most houses were left empty, livestock without owners, lands uncultivated, fruits and crops left to spoil, children abandoned and orphaned. Families were wiped out, the living doubled over with trials and miseries, curates tenuous, the mines without workers,

7. Ovid, *Metamorphoses* 7.602: "Ante sacros vidi projecta cadaver a postes."

governors facing many losses and setbacks, royal tributes diminished. The well and the contaminated suffered equal calamity in all but the benefit of life, which is incomparable.

Not a single [religious] image was less than encumbered with promises, nor a single saint without payment for a special cult, imploring its patronage, and in particular those helpful patrons in times of plague: Saint Sebastian, Saint Anthony Martyr, Saint Roch, Saint John Sahagún, and others, with sung masses, devout novenas, and reverent obsequies of candles and adornments in their arches. And once again the diocesan council swore in on September 16, as patron and advocate of the epidemics, Saint Francis Xavier, obliging all to observe his feast day each year in the Jesuit church, attending in the form of the whole city and under maces, the vote for which was accepted the following day by the father rector Luis de Necolalde. The prebend holders also swore to Saint Roch, but without the same solemnity, as done by the Apostolic See.

At the high point of mortality, which came at the end of July, there was seen on Friday, the twenty-sixth of the same month, at night, toward the north, many fiery exhalations like those of the year 1683, called by modern philosophers night lights or aurora borealis, which rise up from time to time in the form of plumes, like a bonfire, all of which added no small terror to the laments and afflictions in which the city found itself. It lasted half an hour.

Aside from the pestiferous and variable air, the vapor was still more pernicious, putrid from so many cadavers and from the clothing of the contaminated thrown into the streets and plazas, such that all became like rubbish heaps, so infectious that one could not walk through them without the antidotes and preservative remedies that medicine recommends for such cases. The city council named, on October 2, deputies for the cathedral chapters and scribes, that they should get the streets cleaned, as they were filled with trash, strips of clothing, and the blankets of the plague-ridden.

According to the most conservative computation and conjecture, there died twenty thousand persons in this city [of Cuzco], and in the provinces and towns of the bishopric up to forty thousand, including Spaniards, Indians, and children, in all sixty thousand, with little error, although some say it surpassed eighty thousand, as there was no exact numeration nor calculation due to the general confusion. But it is no small blow, sixty thousand, to such a thin population as there is in this province. This fatal and formidable destruction caused such horror that even hyperbole fell short. Everything was a continuous somersault, with men going about engrossed and riled, unable to concentrate on their actions and business dealings, finding themselves possessed by the terror. At the very peak of the plague, so hardened now by so much evil, the eyes grew dry and unable to produce tears, which the physicians count among the symptoms and signs of pestilence. And thus there ceased the mourning even upon burying the dead, but also because there was no one around to mourn. Oedipus offered the same complaint:

> Rather, the persistent devastation of so much evil
> Has itself drained our eyes dry: because as often happens in
>     extreme situations,
> Our tears have perished.[8]

And of the Myrmidons, [according to] Ovid:

> Those who would cry are gone.[9]

In great misfortunes mourning is typically consoling, calming the afflicted heart, a comfort amid sorrows, remedy for sadness, and relief from burdens.

"Weeping lightens one's woes," as [Ulysses] said.[10]

But (oh what pain!) the most lamentable thing of all was the hardness of souls (please permit me this as an apostrophe), as these mortals, asleep in their vices, and their consciences plagued in the midst of such calamity, the same that excited the mercy of the Lord, yet they did not mend their ways, nor did quarrels cease, nor thefts, nor frauds, nor scandals, nor injustices, nor other iniquities among the white folk [gente blanca], but rather they carried on with greater

---

8. Seneca, *Oedipus* 57–59 (from Oedipus's opening monologue): "Quin ispa tanti pervicax clades mali / Siccavit oculos: quod quem extremis solet / periere lacrimae."
    9. Ovid, *Metamorphoses* 7.611: "Qui lacriment desunt, etc."
    10. Seneca, *Trojan Women* 765 (Ulysses speaking to Andromache, who has asked her captor for time to mourn her son, Astyanax): "Fletus ærumnas levat."

vehemence, using up the time God had conceded them in gambling and other frivolities, such that these had never been more frequent in this city.

The Indians carried on with their own abuses, claiming to see various apparitions and shades. In particular, they said that an ancient beggar, a pilgrim, came from the province of Collao all the way to Cuzco with the name of Plague, threatening each town, the same as happened in that [pandemic] of the year 1589, as one reads in the Jesuits' annual letters. In places they went beyond superstitious observance, as was discovered in a village in the parish of Saint Jerome, where they worshipped the Common Enemy, whose effigy they had painted on paper. And at one point, when they were celebrating their diabolical rites, they were discovered in this abominable exercise by Fray José de Azpilcueta of the Order of Preachers, companion of the priest of that rural parish, and he punished them severely, as they deserved, for such a grave and furthermore inexcusable crime, and he took the image of that accursed swindler, which was displayed by Fray Gabriel Romero of the same order, relating the whole case in a sermon he gave in this city on a Thursday night, July 25, in the Jesuit church.

There were also observed many strange occurrences, such as the fact that many of those contaminated got well after certain chance actions, some by bathing in cold water, which they threw themselves into in the heat of fever, others for having drunk it, and there were even some who, placed in the cemetery, recovered and remained well. It occurred on September 8 in the cathedral that one buried body, among others from the day before, placed near the plinth and cordon of the altar of Our Lady of La Antigua, stuck out the greater part of an arm, reaching above the surface of the pavement. It was one of those [cadavers] looked after by Dr. don Félix Cortés, attorney for the royal audiencia of Lima and rector of this church [the Cuzco cathedral], who from five or six steps away said, "That arm is calling me." And that same day he contracted the illness, from which he died on the fifteenth [of September].

They recovered the hand and covered it with substantial earth, but the next day, ninth of the said month, they again found it outside. And now with certain care they put it back again, covering it with more dirt, and in order to hold it down better they placed on top of it a square stone block. And yet, in spite of this weight, they saw the next day, the tenth, that it had come out again, the block to one side. The whole thing remained a mystery, no one knowing what it could be, nor even what body it [the arm or hand] belonged to, but they did not investigate further since later a cleric, ordering it cut off, had it thrown into a pit in the cemetery.

At the beginning of November, the overall strength of the fever began to decline, and, as the rains picked up, it ceased altogether, Glory to God! [but] leaving behind lamentable memories to posterity. It was exactly seventy years after the great earthquakes of 1650, and it was called the Gran Peste. There continued a general scarcity of food for two years, not due to the sterility of the land or lack of rain but for the lack of Indians, the only ones who work the land in agriculture. Due to the shortage in this year of 1720, they lost most of the harvest, unable to store anything in the granaries. The general and common decline and disruption that this epidemic caused in royal tributes, in property values, and in other means of human living in all this kingdom, is quite notorious, and it took many years to recover. And now, enough with the sad memories; let us plead with the Lord, who sends these tribulations by his infinite mercy.

# 3

## Apocalypse in Arequipa

*Our closest equivalent source from Arequipa, a sun-splashed city in Peru's southern highlands, is by the priest Ventura Travada y Córdova (1695–1758). "Travada," as he is remembered, penned a history of his hometown in the year 1750 under the curious title* The Soil of Arequipa Converted into Heaven.[1] *The manuscript blends genres, beginning with volcanic eruptions and ending with a shower of sonnets and epigrams, with histories of the city's convents and churches plus a hagiography of its bishops sandwiched in between.*

*Travada says the city of Arequipa, not counting the Indigenous villages and enslaved African-staffed vineyards around it, was home to about thirty thousand people in 1750, perhaps four thousand of them Indigenous. The 1719 population may have been similar, but likely with a higher Indigenous proportion. More like Potosí's Arzáns than Cuzco's Esquivel, Travada emphasizes what he calls "prodigies," or inexplicable events that seem to be either God's or the devil's handiwork. In one case from the 1680s, a dazed and confused Spaniard appears magically on the slopes of Misti Volcano. Rescued by an Indigenous herder, he is brought to town convinced he was teleported directly from Seville. Travada believes it.*

*Like Esquivel and Arzáns, Travada treats the Gran Peste of 1719–20 as both an extreme event and as one of a string of tragedies, yet another inscrutable divine judgment, like pirate attacks, earthquakes, droughts, and volcanic eruptions. For Travada, the plague is set in the context of the tenure of Arequipa bishop Juan de Otálora Bravo de Laguna, who died a few years later, in 1723. Thus, it serves as a character test, which he ably passes. Of the plague's thousands of victims, we learn next to nothing.*

### S.XV[2]

Carrying on with the same life of this lord bishop [Otálora], there disembarked in Buenos Aires an English ship with a cargo of Blacks, and [it] being a vessel blown by the cold Aquilon [wind], one could

---

1. See Galdos Rodríguez, *Cronistas e historiadores*, 87–132.
2. Travada y Córdova, *Suelo de Arequipa*.

not hope for anything good to come of it, and, serving as ballast to that ship, there came one of the cruelest plagues ever seen in this world, such that in sinking into this extremely vast kingdom it killed more than the third part of its people, still without its contagion having reached its cities and the western towns of the seacoast, and the majority of those who died were Indians, Blacks, and their mixtures and less so the Spaniards.

In their "gentile-hood," as they live in the jungles of the Montaña [i.e., Amazonia], it has been said that certain Chunchos, in order to explain the great number of people who among them died, had no more proper language with which to explain than to toss a fistful of dirt in the air, wanting it to be understood that the dead were innumerable, like grains of sand. The device of this universal infirmity was a catarrh, with many relapses, and most expelling blood through the nostrils, but with so many variations that its symptoms were incomprehensible to the most skillful physicians, and with those [remedies] that healed some, others died.

They said that it was an effect of a great solar eclipse that occurred in the year 1718 [*sic*, 1719] on August 15, during which the solar disc was completely blacked out for three hours, and in many parts of the kingdom those three hours of that day were a most gloomy night. To me (although I have been a rigid skeptic of astrological aphorisms), it makes me doubt that in the pontifical [histories] there is no mention of a similar plague that also had as prelude an eclipse in every way similar to the aforementioned.

Before this plague arrived in this city, the most illustrious [bishop] went out to visit his bishopric (and not to flee the plague, as one rival ordered it printed in a gazette), and, being out there visiting the [northwest] provinces of Collahuas and Condesuyos with news that the plague had entered the city, he ordered his majordomo, who remained in Arequipa, to succor the sick with generous and continuous alms, not withholding any income, and so that this mandate should have the exact complement to that gifted by the charity of His Illustriousness, and of all common necessities, he gave an order that all the confessors and physicians of the city, taking account of the needs of those whom they went out to confess, that they draw up credit slips, assigning the quantities as needed to aid the sick.

And at the instant that they received the order, the confessors and physicians began to dispatch the money orders to the [bishop's] palace at all hours and for various amounts according to the requirements of the needy, and like exhalations and vapors that by the attraction of the sun rise to the appropriate region and return to enrich the earth, filling the canals to the brim and [providing] bountiful harvests, thus those promissory notes, which by the power of the sun of charity rose to the heavens of the episcopal palace, informing it, these vapors and exhalations of the pestilential fever, returned raining down as generous and continuous succor to all the infirmaries, filling them with relief for their cures and victuals.

But harried by so many alms, the majordomo wrote to His Illustriousness to give a new order, as already in such a short time there had been spent 40,000 pesos, and the need was rising with the plague, and in a short time the palace would be left without income even for basic necessities. Great was the sorrow that His Illustriousness felt to see the majority of his flock amid the flames of the plague, but that day it tempered its sentiment with the news that he gave to the majordomo, to whom he wrote again that, no matter what he had spent, to go on distributing alms in the same manner, and that God would never falter, and if by chance he should come up short of money and for all his efforts he could not search it out, he should sell everything he had, not even reserving the pontifical and the pectorals [i.e., his bejeweled personal effects], and if by chance he will have come to have sold them to succor the needs [of the people] it would be the most delightful news he could receive in his whole life.

*Travada goes on to say that Bishop Otálora later sold a prized piece of unicorn horn set in gold given to him by a prelate in Cuzco. Better to give away this antidote, he said, than to keep it and "poison his conscience."*

*Other Arequipa pandemic narratives are of later vintage, some collected and digested around the year 1800 by Basque cleric Juan Domingo Zamácola y Jáuregui. Influenced by his own times and vocabulary, Zamácola adopts a dispassionate tone. Even so, he seems to quote directly from sources composed nearer to the time of the Gran Peste.[3]*

3. Polo, *Apuntes sobre las epidemias*, 28–31. Polo cites the priest Juan Domingo Zamácola y Jáuregui (b. 1746 in Dima, Bizkaya), founder of the parish of Caima. As Arequipa's first major historian, Zamácola wrote *Apuntes para la historia de Arequipa*, circa 1800. See also Barriga, *Terremotos en Arequipa*, 292. Polo also cites Cateriano, *Memorias de los Ilmos*, 160. Another source suggested that, in all, a third of Arequipa's Spanish population died, along with two-thirds of its Indigenous population. The "corrupt" south winds were said to have altered peoples' humors and the "mass," or consistency, of their blood. See Echeverría, *Memoria de la Santa Iglesia*, 4:47. Polo, *Apuntes sobre las epidemias*, also quotes Echeverría on page 30, but without a citation.

In the months of July, August, and September [1719], there were observed in Arequipa some very hot and extremely fetid south winds, which right away gave occasion to the most alert to fear fatal consequences. The heaviness and thickness of the winds corrupted the atmosphere, and within a short time there was felt the contagion of the plague, which spread very quickly, such that by the end of September there was not a subject great or small in the city and its environs that remained untouched by the illness. The streets and plazas were left deserted, it being only a rare individual that one saw walking through them. Provisions ran short, as there was no one to bring them to market nor anyone to send out to buy them, and thus amid the confusion normal subsistence and attentiveness disappeared.

The sickness consisted of a great heaviness and faintness of the head, weakness of all the senses, the body aching indistinctly in all its parts, general lassitude, deafness and a total despondency and lack of appetite, bleeding from the mouth and nose, plus fever. Those who suffered chronic illnesses, especially of the chest, died instantly, and the same happened to those who, following the advice of physicians, had their blood let. Those of good constitution found some relief by using sweating agents and heavy covers to encourage transpiration. Convalescence was very drawn out and belabored, as the body remained so weak, the vision cloudy, the aspect and will depressed, the remnants of the affliction requiring much time to dissipate.

The greater part of the city was left deserted, there being so many dead that the churches and cemeteries could not take them. To help out, some large carts were built to transport the bodies out to the countryside, where they were given burial in some great trenches ordered dug for the purpose. The houses of the city were for the most part left open, and many of them totally abandoned, no one taking the least care for their valuables and furniture. But the destruction felt in the valleys and small towns around the city was much greater, really incomparable, especially in Puquina Canyon, which was totally desolate. . . .

The bishop of Arequipa, [Juan Bravo] Otálora, rescued the poor with all his income from loans he took out, and he even reached the point of selling his furniture and pectoral [i.e., bejeweled cross] for the remediation of common needs.

# 4

---

## Signs and Symptoms

*In 1723 viceregal court physician Federico Bottoni (1669–1745), a native of Messina, Sicily, published a short treatise in Lima titled* Evidence of the Circulation of Blood. *Dr. Bottoni had been a practicing physician in the household of the queen of Spain in Madrid between 1701 and 1714, when the young monarch, Maria Luisa of Savoy, succumbed to tuberculosis. Bottoni made his way to Peru around 1715, where, in addition to treating viceroys and rich locals, he served as book inspector and interpreter for the Holy Office of the Inquisition.*

*That Bottoni was respected is evidenced by a laudatory foreword by Dr. Pedro Peralta Barnuevo, Lima's most learned man and rector of the University of San Marcos. In a section of his short book describing his special treatments for smallpox, including deer horn, bezoar stones, and similar substances, Bottoni turns to the "famous plague" that shook all of greater Peru, but especially the highlands, just as he was composing his work.[1] He provides a rare description of the disease's symptoms as they progressed day by day.*

Which leads us to say, and with such painful clauses, we may with squinted eyes explain the horrible and wretched devastations of the famous plague, which with equal tyranny has run a thousand and more leagues from Buenos Aires all the way to the outskirts of Lima without letting up with its fatal cruelty but rather more furious, not only against the lives of the greater part of the Indians, but it also no longer spares the Spaniard, the mestizo, nor the Black, laying waste equally to the whole country, and one who manages to free oneself from its fatal insults in the end succumbs to a painful death by hunger.

---

1. This section is from Bottoni, *Evidencia*, fols. 22v–23v, n.p. The literature on Peralta Barnuevo is vast. See Hill, *Sceptres and Sciences*, chap. 3. Hill also discusses Bottoni in some depth on pages 163–64.

The multiplicity of signs and symptoms produced by this monstrous plague is due to a mortal venom, which is extremely corrosive and variable, and with great force and speed it disturbs spirits, consuming them, corrupting the fibers [i.e., thickening agents] of the liquids, which quickly run impetuously with free rein, their channels unable to contain them, and finally the same solid substances, transmuted, prove the ferocity of the root cause.

We have witnessed the effects of the invincible force of this poison, not far from Lima, in the [house of the] Discalced Recollects of Saint Mary of the Angels in the Alameda [and in the person] of an exemplary religious, the father Fray Domingo Arbolea, *montañés* [mountaineer], who more than three months earlier had left Cajamarca, the affliction having passed through all parts of the Sierra, for the most part plague-ridden.

Within four days of having arrived, on February 20, [1721?], he came down with a light fever, which he tolerated standing. But the second day was truly awful, with great debility and pains all over the body, and the third day he suffered the same unease. On the fourth day his fever rose and his chest heaved, there appearing the fatal blood from the mouth, with the body aches continuing, more severe on the left side, the respiration belabored with a bit of a rattle. The fifth day the fatigues were no greater, but on the sixth day all the symptoms grew more pronounced, and he totally lost his remaining strength, and with a mildly cold sweat he gave his soul to God, in all, six days of a truly pestilential illness.

In all this one observed the general weakening, the shortness [or mildness] of the fever on the surface, the urine good, but the blood totally altered in color, without substance [*sin fibras*], and the sputum bloodied, but showing upon closer examination something like pieces of the lung, corrupted, the pain always continuing with greater force, and lastly [the symptoms of] this illness seemed to be exacerbated every other day.

One could offer many reflections on this particular case and on the "Sierra plague" more broadly, but right now the brevity of my role does not permit me to extend into digressions, however useful.

*Bottoni ends by recommending a treatise on the disease by one Dr. don Manuel de Alcibia, a former mathematics professor at the University of Mexico currently practicing as a physician in Guamanga (today Ayacucho, Peru), "who as eyewitness has painted the horrible monster with great priority and diligence."[2]*

The famous Peruvian physician and scientist Hipólito Unanue (1755–1833), writing around the turn of the nineteenth century, referred back to Bottoni and others in his discussion of the great pestilence of 1719–20.[3] Unanue could not help but claim that the August 15, 1719, solar eclipse was in fact a harbinger of the pandemic although, as we have seen, earlier authors tended to see it as a contributing factor but not a cause. Unanue cites Peralta Barnuevo, who (as Arzáns noted) considered the eclipse significant. Unanue also cites Travada on Arequipa, ending his brief description of Peru's Gran Peste with classical references linking it to human vanity.

2. I have been unable to locate this work.
3. Unanue, *Observaciones sobre el clima*, 25, 124.

# 5

## The Cure

*Indigenous Andeans were the principal victims of the great Andean pandemic of 1717–22, followed, it seems, by a significant number of enslaved Africans and their descendants plus a number of mixed and Spanish, Portuguese, or otherwise European poor folk, and yet we have virtually no idea of what therapies were applied. Presumably, some of those infected were fortunate enough to receive palliative care. For the vast majority there was no known cure, only the hope that bloodletting or violent purges would not make things worse.*

*One physician's claim of having discovered a cure for the Gran Peste appears in a letter sent anonymously from Cuzco to medical authorities in Lima. It seems to date from late 1720, and in it we learn more about European medical theories and proposed remedies than about Indigenous ones. Even so, the author provides rare insight on an Andean therapy, a bitter bean known in English as lupine, along with the physician's own proposed cure, either blessed thistle or a local substitute, similar to safflower and common in the central Andes.*

*The anonymous physician also recommends a strict diet, followed to match the course of the symptoms described in the previous chapter. How many patients were saved by thistle and safflower we do not know, but our anonymous author suspects that many were killed by the false remedies of lupine (too hot and dry) and quince juice (too astringent).*

*The author was addressing a high-ranking contemporary medical authority in Lima, the royal protomédico or "surgeon general," Dr. Bernabé Ortiz de Landaeta. Ortiz also emphasized the importance of diet and its alleged connection to disease susceptibility in his report to King Philip V, but in a different context. Diet was more preventative than curative in this view. Based on a variety of reports but no known firsthand observations, Ortiz claimed that the Gran Peste had started in Buenos Aires in 1717 when infected African slaves were exposed to the local poor.*

[Without] a quarantine in place for their disembarkation, with ease this pestilent quality was communicated to everyone in that region pertaining to the lower orders and bottom ranks of the hierarchy, they being the subjects most susceptible to experiencing such high mortality, because being poor they consume those foods we call *multe molis et pauce virtutis* [high bulk, low value] along with noxious beverages, chicha [maize beer], and things of that sort, which almost always disposes them to corruption . . . [whereas] the Spaniards who follow a diet and consume the foods we call *multe virtutis et pauce molis* [high value, low bulk] in these regions, it has been rare to find one who has been infected and thus perished.[1]

*This sounds like contempt for the poor, and no surprise. Other observers, including Arzáns and Travada, displayed their disinterest in native Andeans and Africans as individuals in favor of charitable, "heroic" Spaniards. One senses a confluence of racist and classist assumptions, on which grand theories were being constructed or reinforced, all in the name of rational science and imperial raison d'etat.[2] Closer to the ground, perhaps, if no less prejudiced, is the following anonymous physician's report.*

An informative report on the plague, sent from Cuzco[3]

Re: the remedy that has been found to succor the pestilential sickness that afflicts and runs throughout this entire kingdom, striking the Indians more than the Spanish folk, and, as they [i.e., Indigenous Andeans] are of a hotter constitution, dry and toasted [*adusta*] and as the disposition and influences of the air are more analogous to theirs than to [the constitution] of the Spaniards, although they have certainly also been affected, especially those who may have the hot, dry, and toasted constitution.

[With] the conjuncture of Mars and Saturn that we've had for two years, having set in motion great alterations, as much in the air as in human bodies, plus the droughts and heat that have been experienced, it is only to be expected that humans would suffer and more so those who are analogous with the present quality of the stars, the sicknesses of their type, the same that has spread throughout the kingdom, a high, transient fever that results in toasted, melancholic blood, so violent that it destroys the miserable person in an instant,

1. Transcribed in Colin, *Cuzco*, 38n34 (my translation). I thank Prof. Gabriela Ramos for pointing me to this source and Michael Brumbaugh for translations from the Latin.
2. See Earle, *Body of the Conquistador*.
3. The report is taken from the transcription of a portion of AGI, Lima 411, by Colin, *Cuzco*, 187–91. Colin titles the appendix "Piece Justificative, No. 1."

as is known from the deaths and destruction it has caused from Buenos Aires to here.

It all [i.e., the cure] has to do with the virtue of bitterness, though not quite astringent, as out of bitterness comes the virtue of correcting the choleric humor, softening its sharpness and fieriness, retarding the fermentation, which is what produces corruption and death, separating from the mass of blood the poisonous and hidden contagion, which has been taken in from the corrupt air, [the cure] quitting thirst, exciting the appetite, and by its penetration carrying [the poison] off by way of the urine, until the symptoms end in health and the ill person is rescued as they should be, comforting the heart and providing them robustness so as not to absorb the contagion—and in the end quitting and separating the plague from human bodies.

So it is written by Dr. Mena [Fernando de Mena, 1520–85] in his treatise on pestilential fever, folio 45 . . . Virgil teaches us the same, exalting the virtue of cider as cure for the plague. . . . A proof of these doctrines, especially that of Dr. Mena: *modo non astringant* [now nonrestrictive] is that the juice of quince has been the [fatal] knife, since by its coldness, dryness, and restriction [i.e., astringency] it has destroyed so many people by impeding transpiration, trapping the poison in the most noble and principal parts of the body, which it annihilates by not allowing exit, utterly destroying [the body] and occasioning death. The same is said by the extremely wise Heredia [Pedro Miguel Heredia, 1579–1655] on the curing of malignant fever, vol. 5, fol. 615 . . . and thus it is known that more people may have died from quince juice that was given improperly than from the illness itself.

It should be noted in the same way that *chochos* have been no remedy in this pestilential illness, as has been experienced, since, if taken as bitters, from their bitterness it has been seen that they kill [intestinal] worms, which the ill have expelled from the mouth and bowels, without recognizing in them [the chochos] any pharmacological virtue that might oppose the violence of the pestilence, as has been experienced here.[4] It is an evident proof that they have been of no

4. Chochos (*Lupinus mutabilis*), or "lupine seeds," are a kind of Andean bean known in Quechua as *tarwi*. They are listed in a circa 1636 "medical shopping list" for recently arrived African slaves in Lima; see Newson and Minchin, *From Capture to Sale*, 265. Current experiments with bitter alkaloids in Andean lupine suggest they are effective against intestinal worms in ruminants. The author of our remedy from 1720 seems to suggest that unleached lupine seeds were taken as a folk remedy for the great Andean peste since they were demonstrably effective in this way as vermicide.

use to those who have taken them, as the majority of those who have received them to get well have perished. Without doubt it is because the said chochos are of a hot and dry temperament, and with this temperament they have irritated the hottest material (cause of the illness) and added to its heat, causing the violent fermentation of the blood and greater putrefaction, and as a result a quicker death, even if it brings about the expulsion of worms, as they are not the cause of the illness that must be attended to.

If the sick are in a state ready to take drink after the fever has broken and symptoms ceased, [it is better to avoid] the effects of medicines, which for their bitterness, heat, and innate properties might destroy worms, as they may do harm by augmenting the illness as the said chochos have done.

And it is settled doctrine that during fevers, if there is found a case of worms, they are not to be cured by giving medicines to destroy them, especially hot ones, because they cause the ill to perish. So it is said by Guillermo Rondelacio [Guillaume Rondelet of Montpellier, 1507–66] in his treatise on medicine, fol. 476 . . . [And these are all] reasons that prove the inappropriateness of bitter chochos, and from them there may have died an infinite number of Indians in the highlands. Because given that they possess the virtue of killing worms that is attributed to them only for being bitter, for being hot and dry they oppose the quality and malignity of the fever, [allowing that] it being certain that with time [what] could be an antidote is without it [i.e., sufficient time] poisonous.

And it is evident that there is nothing found in chochos that could oppose the pestilence. Rather, one finds in blessed thistle all that may be directed to the desired end, as it has the virtue of resistance, opposing itself to the plague and separating it from the body while [also] destroying and annihilating the worms, alleviating and quitting the pain of the abdomen, which as a symptom or effect of this poisonous contagion often takes the lives of the most wretched among the sick.[5] And it is so efficacious that [on my] having given it to only a few of them, they have experienced total relief, and they have been freed from the plague, without such heat that we may be astonished, since the means of administering it, as will be declared, could not cause the least harm to the sick but should rather give them all consolation.

5. Blessed thistle (*Cnicus benedictus*) is a Mediterranean plant used to treat plague.

Thus it is written by Andrés Mathiolo [Pietro Andrea Mattioli of Siena, 1501–77] in his comment on Dioscorides, fol. 167 of the second volume, . . . to these remedies one must add the scarlet pimpernel and chicory, vulgarly called *pillipilli* in the Incaic language [i.e., Quechua], deer antler filed or grated, placed in a clean cloth, tied up and boiled with its wrappings, as they do for those poor sick ones, with pomegranate juice or in a syrup, if it can be found, so as to recalibrate [*corroborar*] the heart. And because I understand that it would not be very easy to find everywhere and less so in the *puna* [i.e., high-altitude desert], the abundance of blessed thistle necessary to treat such a multitude of sick people, as it is barely found in this city [of Cuzco] in flowerpots and in some gardens kept out of curiosity by certain persons on behalf of the physicians, they could take advantage of another herb of the same species as blessed thistle, which could serve as substitute and fill in for its absence and which has the same properties, temperaments, and virtues.

And this is what out of ignorance certain healers [*curanderos*], who come to these regions without knowledge of the plants, call black salsify, wanting to reduce to clear proof of verifiable cures that which a sick person has carried by chance and to apply it to all manner of constitutions, this single remedy, while ignoring its specific properties and means of acting on a person's natural balance, it being certain that in this faculty it is not right to practice without the science of the theoretical, as Plato assures in the axiom that says, *Ars nulla sine ratione* [roughly, "No art without reason"].[6]

Salsify, being quite distinct, as it shows with its makeup [*fábrica*] and flavor, revealing thus its great heat and dryness such that, in my opinion, it is Atractylis [*A. gummifera*, used in Morocco as a medicine] and no other such thing is found anywhere in the *puna*. The physicians of this city [Cuzco] prescribe an infusion of it for malignant fevers, vulgarly called *tabardillos*, being ignorant of their [true] quality. And as such illnesses need to transpire so that the mass of blood may free itself of the poison that has it oppressed and squeezed by the obstructions, most often being the cause of these [symptoms], the medicament enters with its hot virtue to open the pores, making

6. Black salsify (*Scorzonera hispanica*) is a European plant with edible roots, used as an antivenin and plague remedy.

the humors transpire when found to be noxious and opposed to the conservation of the person's nature [i.e., natural balance].

And it is not that [true] salsify would not be an effective medicine for the intended purpose, because all the remedies that serve to defend the human body against external poisons, such as snake bites, are effective in saving it from contagion . . . so says Mathiolo [Mattioli] cited on fol. 491 of vol. 1, and thus the said plant could serve in the way already mentioned. That is all the discussion needed, since what is called for is something that opposes such a violent and contagious illness, providing relief and remedy:

> "For it is generally agreed that a physician should not be long-winded, because illnesses are not repelled by chattering but by the essences or powers of medicines."[7]

I do not recommend here the remedies doctors tout in their treatises against plagues, found only in the hands of pharmacists. First, because the poverty of the Indians means they could not pay for them and, second, because it would be necessary to use them only under direction of physicians, of which there are none in the pueblos, nor would they practice (even if they were available) among the poor, for whom I have procured to direct this succinct and brief method, which I'll discuss, [worthy only] after [His] Divine Mercy, to whom first of all one must appeal to assist all remedies, which here will be given for the common good, especially for the poor, and to his Most Holy Mother, to whom I plead as intercessor, and I beg to reach her son to favor this light discourse. Because if God does not wish to aid it, conferring virtue on the remedies, it is pointless to discuss or put down anything [in writing]. Thus is it said by the most wise Heurnio [Johannes Heurnius of Utrecht, 1543–1601]:

> "Unless God is present and imparts powers to herbs
> What good, I ask, is dittany? What good is panacea?"[8]

---

7. "Convenit enim Medicum non loquacem, quia morbi non vocibus, sed rerum essentiis, aut viribus repelluntur."

8. "Ni Deus adfuerit, vires que infunderit herbis / Quid rogo dictamnus? quid panacea juvent?"

And moving along toward hope, which we must have in God
for all things, without whose aid medicines have no effect and with
whose charge one sees remedies succeed, the same author continues,

"The only safe bet for the sick is to not give up on salvation,
The only safe bet is that no one can hope for salvation without
God."[9]

This understood, the cure should take the following form: as soon
as someone falls ill with the plague, which is evidenced by chills after
a high fever, headache, the heart afflicted, and the pulse pounding the
first day, at first rapid, then slow and weak, though elevated in some,
and in others who do not feel feverish only feel the heart, which
afflicts them, such that they have a desire to vomit, adding stomachaches and abdominal pains, the appetite destroyed, an insatiable
thirst, sandpaper tongue, or [the tongue] stained black or "juicy,"
depending on where the poison is located, which may or may not
send soot to the mouth and tongue, staining it.

One may prescribe ordinary palliatives [ayudas], with infusions
of mallow, bran, and chamomile in small quantities, with a cut of beef
cooked in ordinary water, the same strained after being well boiled;
one should add a piece of unsalted hunto [untu? Quechua for llama
fat], six ounces of sugar, the brownest one can find, and a touch of
salt, and these palliatives administered the first day in order to exon-
erate the person's natural balance, which will last to the next day, on
which others will be administered for the subsequent three days, first
afternoon, then morning, in the following manner:

Take a good cut of beef; a handful of mallow; a handful of
thyme; four or five leaves of borage; a lettuce, if available and,
if not, it is of little importance; half a sleeve of chamomile; a
handful of rose, which, if not available, is again of no matter.

Put it all together and cook in putrid urine, and, after it is good
and boiling, one should add as only one extra palliative measure

9. "Una salus aegris non desperare salutem, / Una salus nullem absque Deo
sperare salutem."

[*malagón*] of vinegar, four ounces of brown sugar, or that which is available.

This is to be administered until the fourth day, and, having passed into the fifth, one must take four to six leaves of blessed thistle, and, if it is not to hand, then the aforementioned salsify [*escorzonera*], and sew it up in a pouch, well mashed, in a jug of water, and, after squeezing and straining the pouch, if there is still much fever and thirst [in the patient], one expresses into the said remedy the juice of half a lime and, if unavailable, a tablespoon of good vinegar with a bit of sugar, to be given to the sick person while fasting, repeating this in the late evening, and more if the [sick] one is found to have stomachaches and abdominal pain, which mortally afflicts the plague-stricken in this case we are now experiencing, taking their lives even faster than the violence of the fever, and one continues until the pain and fever subsides, so as afterward to continue with only borage [infusion] afternoon and morning until [the patient] seems fully restored, because borage tempers and expels the poison that has been extracted from the blood by the remedy of the bitters.

Start also from the first day until after the fourth to drink water boiled in chicory or scarlet pimpernel with deer antler filed or grated, and, in the pouch made for each drink, one should mix in half a tablespoon of vinegar plus another half [tablespoon] of bitter cider or, if not [available], lemon, with its sugar, drinking the said compound afternoon and morning as has been prescribed, so as to then move on to the blessed thistle treatment.

All this must be carried out, and in those places where one finds no limes or cider, the only thing needed is vinegar.

And, after [the patient] seems better, it may come to pass that one finds oneself with a certain weakness of the stomach occasioned by the continuation of the bitters, one may, if the fever has died down, drink water boiled with a bulb of fennel or some chamomile flowers with a bit of sugar so as to repair [*componer*] the stomach if needed. If a pomegranate is available, consider adding a few tablespoons of its juice. After the [patient's symptoms] are alleviated, use just the borage as prescribed.

This cure is most certain and secure if one attempts to feed the plague-stricken, and more so this plague that has spread, as it is known that the sick in a single day can be wiped out and consumed, rendered corrupt with such strange brevity that it is said the same thing could happen with a hectic [i.e., spiking] fever, without which one might allege that in an impure body the more you feed it, the more it injures and mistreats itself:

> "Impure bodies, the more you nourish them, the more you harm them."[10]

And thus Galen says in 3 *Epidem.* comm. 3, test. 98,[11] that, in the plague of his time, the sick had such an abhorrence for food that for lack of it they all perished, and for those whom they force-fed against their will, all survived, and only those who refused food died:

> "In the time of Galen's plague, there was so much aversion to and abomination of food that many were saying that they would prefer to die than to eat, and all were set free who forced themselves to eat."[12]

In all the foods [administered] try to add vinegar or lime. And because the great amount of blood that tends to come out of the mouths and noses of the suffering tends to be copious and violent, so much so that it often takes their lives, if by chance you come upon them at the first instance, without them having experienced fever, right after you see them eject the said blood, give them to drink a measure [*malagón*] of cold vinegar with a piece of milled sugar, also applying to the [abdomen?] the said vinegar mixed with starch or milled white maize and also to the nose, repeating this until the remedy slows it down [i.e., the bloody ejections], and after it has been detained you move on to the cure as prescribed, and if during the curing process the blood should flow again, one should perform the same application.

And it should be known that bloodletting for this ailment is opposed and pernicious, and although one may according to judgment contain the blood, which may be by diversion, which in that case would be done in the ankle, it should be done only in very small

---

10. "Impura corpora quo plus nutris es magis ledis."

11. The reference is to Galen's *Commentary* on the Hippocratic *Epidemics.*

12. "In temore pestis Galeni tanta era ciborum aversio, / Et abominatio quod multi dicebant se velle prius mori, / Quam comedere et qui vim sibi afferentes comedebant, / Omnes liberati fuerant."

amounts according to necessity, although it has been shown that many have been healed with only that prescribed earlier, without any bleeding at all. God disposes in all that which most pleases him, and may it be for the good of all.

Alchon, Suzanne Austin. *A Pest in the Land: New World Epidemics in a Global Perspective*. Albuquerque: University of New Mexico Press, 2003.

Arcondo, Aníbal. "Mortalidad general, mortalidad epidémica, y comportamiento de la población de Córdoba durante el siglo XVIII." *Desarrollo Económico* 33, no. 129 (1993): 67–85.

Arzáns de Orsúa y Vela, Bartolomé. *Historia de la Villa Imperial de Potosí*. Edited by Gunnar Mendoza and Lewis Hanke. 3 vols. Providence: Brown University Press, 1965.

Bakewell, Peter. *Silver and Entrepreneurship in Seventeenth-Century Potosí: The Life and Times of Antonio López de Quiroga*. Albuquerque: University of New Mexico Press, 1988.

Barragán, Rossana. "Ladrones, pequeños empresarios, o trabajadores independientes? K'ajchas, trapiches, y plata en el Cerro Rico de Potosí en el siglo XVIII." *Nuevo Mundo / Mundos Nuevos* (2015). https://journals.openedition.org/nuevomundo/67938.

———. "Working Silver for the World: Mining Labor and Popular Economy in Colonial Potosí." *Hispanic American Historical Review* 97, no. 2 (2017): 193–222.

Barriga, Victor. *Los terremotos en Arequipa*. Arequipa, Peru: Colmena, 1951.

Bertrand, Jean-Baptiste. *A Historical Relation of the Plague at Marseille in the Year 1720*. Translated by Anne Plumptre. London, 1805.

Biedma, José Juan, ed. *Acuerdos del extinguido cabildo de Buenos Aires*. 2nd ser., vol. 3, nos. 16–17 (1714–18). Reprint, Buenos Aires: Archivo General de la Nación, 1926.

Borucki, Alex. "From Asiento to Spanish Networks: Slave Trading in the Río de la Plata, 1700–1810." In *From the Galleons to the Highlands: Slave Trade Routes in the Spanish Americas*, edited by Alex Borucki, David Eltis, and David Wheat, 177–200. Albuquerque: University of New Mexico Press, 2020.

Bottoni, Federico. *Evidencia de la circulación de la sangre*. Lima: Ignacio de Luna, 1723.

Bowers, Kristy Wilson. *Plague and Public Health in Early Modern Seville*. Rochester: University of Rochester Press, 2013.

Carlin, Claire L., ed. *Imagining Contagion in Early Modern Europe*. New York: Palgrave, 2005.

Carrière, Charles. *Marseille, ville mort: La peste de 1720*. Marseille: Garçon, 1968.

Cateriano, Mariano. *Memorias de los Ilmos: SS Obispos de Arequipa*. Arequipa, Peru, 1908.

Celton, Dora Estela. "Enfermedad y crisis de mortalidad en Córdoba, Argentina, entre los siglos XVI y XX." *Cambios demográficos en América Latina: La experiencia de cinco siglos*, 277–99. Córdoba, Argentina: Universidad Nacional de Córdoba, 1998.

Cipolla, Carlo. *Fighting the Plague in Seventeenth-Century Italy*. Madison: University of Wisconsin Press, 1981.

Colin, Michèle. *Le Cuzco à la fin du XVIIe et au début du XVIIIe siècle*. Paris: Editions de l'Institut des Hautes Études de l'Amérique Latine, 1966.

Cook, Alexandra Parma, and Noble D. Cook. *The Plague Files: Crisis Management in Sixteenth-Century Seville*. Baton Rouge: Louisiana State University Press, 2009.

Cook, Noble D. *Born to Die: Disease and New World Conquest, 1492–1650*. New York: Cambridge University Press, 1998.

Cook, Noble D., and George Lovell, eds. *Secret Judgments of God: Old World Epidemics in Colonial Spanish America*. Norman: University of Oklahoma Press, 1991.

Dell, Melissa. "The Persistent Effects of Peru's Mining Mita." *Econometrica* 78, no. 6 (2010): 1863–903.

Dobrizhoffer, Martin. *An Account of the Abipones, an Equestrian People of Paraguay*. Translated by Sara Coleridge. 2 vols., 1784. Reprint, London: Murray, 1822.

———. *Historia de los abipones*. 2 vols. Resistencia, Argentina: Universidad Nacional del Nordeste, 1968.

Dobyns, Henry. "An Outline of Andean Epidemic History to 1720." *Bulletin of the History of Medicine* 37, no. 6 (1963): 493–515.

Eamon, William. "Cannibalism and Contagion: Framing Syphilis in Counter-Reformation Italy." *Early Science and Medicine* 3, no. 1 (1998): 1–31.

Earle, Rebecca. *The Body of the Conquistador: Food, Race and the Colonial Experience in Spanish America, 1492–1700*. New York: Cambridge University Press, 2012.

Echeverría, Francisco Xavier. *Memoria de la Santa Iglesia de Arequipa*, in *Memorias para la historia de Arequipa*. Edited by Víctor Barriga. 4 vols. Arequipa: Editorial La Colmena, 1941–52.

Eckert, Edward A. "The Retreat of Plague from Central Europe, 1640–1720: A Geomedical Approach." *Bulletin of the History of Medicine* 74, no. 1 (2000): 1–28.

Ermus, Cindy. "The Plague of Provence: Early Advances in the Centralization of Crisis Management." *Arcadia: Environment and Society Portal*, no. 9 (2015). Environment and Society. http://www

BIBLIOGRAPHY | 125

.environmentandsociety.org/arcadia/plague-provence-early-advances
-centralization-crisis-management.

———. "The Spanish Plague That Never Was: Crisis and Exploitation in
Cádiz During the Peste of Provence." *Eighteenth-Century Studies* 49,
no. 2 (2016): 167–93.

Esquivel y Navia, Diego de. *Noticias cronológicas de la gran ciudad del
Cuzco*. Edited by Félix Denegri Luna, Horacio Villanueva Urteaga, and
César Gutiérrez Muñoz. 2 vols. Lima: Fundación Wiese, 1980.

Frías, Susana R., and María Inés Montserrat. "Pestes y muerte en el Río de la
Plata y Tucumán (1700–1750)." *Temas de Historia Argentina y Americana* 25, no. 1 (2017): 29–59.

Gaffarel, Paul, and Marquis de Duranty. *La Peste de 1720 a Marseille et en
France d'après des documents inédits*. Paris: Perrin, 1911.

Galdos Rodríguez, Guillermo. *Cronistas e historiadores de Arequipa colonial*.
Arequipa, Peru: Fundación Bustamante de la Fuente / Universidad
Nacional de San Agustín, 1993.

Galeano, Eduardo. *Faces and Masks*. Vol. 2 of *Memory of Fire*. Translated by
Cedric Belfrage. New York: Pantheon, 1987.

Glave, Luis Miguel. "Resistencia y adaptación en una sociedad colonial, el
mundo andino peruano." *Norba* 18 (2005): 51–64.

Hammond, E. Ashby, and Claude Sturgill. "A French Plague Recipe of 1720."
*Bulletin of the History of Medicine* 46, no. 6 (1972): 591–97.

Hanke, Lewis. *Bartolomé Arzáns de Orsúa y Vela's History of Potosí*. Providence: Brown University Press, 1965.

Herrera y Loyzaga, José Cipriano. "Viaje a Buenos Aires, Córdoba, Santiago
de Chile, y Lima en el siglo XVIII (1717–27)." Edited by Guillermo
Furlong. *Historia* 1, no. 2 (1955): 63–80; 1, no. 3 (1956): 135–43.

Hill, Ruth. *Sceptres and Sciences in the Spains: Four Humanists and the
New Philosophy, c. 1680–1740*. Liverpool: Liverpool University Press,
2000.

Inch, Marcela, ed. *Libros de acuerdos del cabildo secular de Potosí*. 5 vols.
Sucre, Bolivia: Archivo y Biblioteca Nacional de Bolivia, 2012.

Jauffret, Louis François. *Pièces historiques sur la peste de Marseille et d'une
partie de la Provence en 1720, 1721, et 1722*. Marseille: Chez les Principaux Libraires, 1820.

Jones, Cameron. *In Service of Two Masters: The Missionaries of Ocopa,
Indigenous Resistance, and Spanish Governance in Bourbon Peru*.
Stanford: Stanford University Press, 2018.

Jones, Colin. "Plague and Its Metaphors in Early Modern France." *Representations* 53 (Winter 1996): 97–127.

Kass, Amalie. "Boston's Historic Smallpox Epidemic." *Massachusetts Historical Review* 14 (2012): 1–51.

Lane, Kris. *Potosí: The Silver City That Changed the World*. Oakland: University of California Press, 2019.

Lanning, John Tate. *The Royal Protomedicato: The Regulation of the Medical Professions in the Spanish Empire.* Edited by John J. TePaske. Durham: Duke University Press, 1985.

Lastres, Juan B. *La medicina en el virreinato.* Vol. 2 of *Historia de la medicina peruana.* Lima: Universidad Nacional Mayor de San Marcos, 1951.

Livi-Bacci, Massimo, and Ernesto J. Maeder. "The Missions of Paraguay: The Demography of an Experiment." *Journal of Interdisciplinary History* 35, no. 2 (2004): 184–224.

Mackay, Ruth. *Life in a Time of Pestilence: The Great Castilian Plague of 1596–1601.* New York: Cambridge University Press, 2019.

Martínez-Vidal, Alvar. *El nuevo sol de la medicina en la Ciudad de los Reyes: Federico Bottoni y la "Evidencia de la circulación de la sangre."* Zaragoza, Spain: Portico, 1990.

Minardi, Margot. "The Boston Inoculation Controversy of 1721–1722: An Incident in the History of Race." *William and Mary Quarterly,* 3rd ser., 61, no. 1 (2004): 47–76.

Molina del Villar, América. *Por voluntad divina: Escasez, epidemias, y otras calamidades en la Ciudad de México, 1700–1762.* Mexico City: Centro de Investigaciones y Estudios Superiores en Antropología Social, 1996.

Moll, Herman, Bernard Lens, and George Vertue. "This Map of South America, According to the Newest and Most Exact Observations." Library of Congress. [1712?]. http://www.loc.gov/item/gm71005444.

Newson, Linda A., and Susie Minchin. *From Capture to Sale: The Slave Trade to Spanish South America in the Early Seventeenth Century.* Leiden, Holland: Brill, 2007.

Palmer, Colin. *Human Cargoes: The British Slave Trade to Spanish America.* Urbana: University of Illinois Press, 1981.

Paul, Helen. *The South Sea Bubble: An Economic History of Its Origin and Consequences.* New York: Routledge, 2011.

Pearce, Adrian. "The Peruvian Population Census of 1725–1740." *Latin American Research Review* 36, no. 3 (2001): 69–104.

Polo, José Toribio. *Apuntes sobre las epidemias en el Perú.* Lima: Barrionuevo, 1913.

Prado, Fabrício. *Anglo-Portuguese Cooperation in Eighteenth-Century Atlantic South America.* New York: Palgrave, forthcoming.

Pueyo, Victor. *Cuerpos plegables: Anatomías de la excepción en España y en América Latina (siglos XVI–XVIII).* Woodbridge, NJ: Boydell, 2016.

Ramírez del Águila, Pedro. *Noticias políticas de Indias y relación descriptiva de la Ciudad de La Plata, metrópoli de las provincias de los Charcas.* Sucre, Bolivia: Ciencia Editores, 2017.

Ramos, Gabriela. *El cuerpo en palabras: Religión, salud, y humanidad en los Andes coloniales.* Lima: Instituto Francés de Estudios Andinos, 2020.

Rivilla Bonet y Pueyo, Joseph de. *Desvíos de la naturaleza o tratado de el origen de los monstros.* Lima: Contreras, 1695.

Sánchez-Albornoz, Nicolás. *Indios y tributos en el Alto Perú*. Lima: Instituto de Estudios Peruanos, 1978.

Santos Guerrero, Fernando. "Epidemias y sublevaciones en el desarrollo demográfico de las misiones Amuesha del Cerro de la Sal, siglo XVIII." *Histórica* 11, no. 1 (1987): 25–53.

Slack, Paul. "Responses to Plague in Early Modern Europe: The Implications of Public Health." *Social Research* 55, no. 3 (1988): 433–53.

Stavig, Ward. *The World of Túpac Amaru: Conflict, Community, and Identity in Colonial Peru*. Lincoln: University of Nebraska Press, 1999.

Suárez, Margarita. *Astros, humores, y cometas: Las obras de Juan Jerónimo Navarro, Joan de Figueroa, y Francisco Ruiz Lozano (Lima, 1645– 1665)*. Lima: Pontificia Universidad Católica del Perú, 2019.

Takeda, Junko Thérèse. *Between Crown and Commerce: Marseille and the Early Modern Mediterranean*. Baltimore: Johns Hopkins University Press, 2011.

Tandeter, Enrique. *Coercion and Market: Silver Mining in Colonial Potosí, 1692–1826*. Translated by Richard Warren. Albuquerque: University of New Mexico Press, 1993.

TePaske, John J. *A New World of Gold and Silver*. Leiden, Holland: Brill, 2010.

Trans-Atlantic Slave Trade Database (year rage: 1715–19; itinerary/principal place of slave landing: Buenos Aires; accessed April 30, 2021). http:// www.slavevoyages.org/voyage/database.

Travada y Córdova, Ventura. *Suelo de Arequipa convertido en cielo*. Edited by Ignacio Prado Pastor. Facsimile ed. Lima: Villanueva, 1993.

Unanue, Hipólito. *Observaciones sobre el clima de Lima y sus influencias en los seres organizados, en especial el hombre*. 2nd ed. Madrid: Imprenta Sancha, 1815.

Varela Peris, Fernando. "El papel de la Junta Suprema de Sanidad en la política sanitaria española del siglo XVIII." *Dynamis* 18 (1998): 315–40.

Vargas Ugarte, Rubén, ed. *Pareceres jurídicos en asuntos de Indias*. Lima: Tipográfica Peruana, 1951.

Voigt, Lisa. *Spectacular Wealth: The Festivals of Colonial South American Mining Towns*. Austin: University of Texas Press, 2016.

Walker, Charles F. *Shaky Colonialism: The 1746 Earthquake-Tsunami in Lima, Peru, and Its Long Aftermath*. Durham: Duke University Press, 2008.

Warren, Adam. *Medicine and Politics in Colonial Peru: Population Growth and the Bourbon Reforms*. Pittsburgh: University of Pittsburgh Press, 2010.

Wightman, Ann M. *Indigenous Migration and Social Change: The Forasteros of Cuzco, 1570–1720*. Durham: Duke University Press, 1990.

Zulawski, Ann. *They Eat from Their Labor: Work and Social Change in Colonial Bolivia*. Pittsburgh: Pittsburgh University Press, 1995.

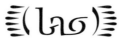

# latin american originals

**Series Editor** | Matthew Restall

This series features primary source texts on colonial and nineteenth-century Latin America, translated into English, in slim, accessible, affordable editions that also make scholarly contributions. Most of these sources are published here in English for the first time and represent an alternative to the traditional texts on early Latin America. The initial focus of the series was on the conquest period in sixteenth-century Spanish America, but its scope now includes later centuries and aims to be hemispheric. LAO volumes feature archival documents and printed sources originally in Spanish, Portuguese, Italian, Latin, Nahuatl, Maya and other Native American languages. The contributing authors are historians, anthropologists, art historians, geographers, and scholars of literature.

Matthew Restall is Edwin Erle Sparks Professor of Latin American History and Anthropology, and Director of Latin American Studies, at the Pennsylvania State University. He edited *Ethnohistory* for a decade and now co-edits the *Hispanic American Historical Review*.

## Board of Editorial Consultants

Kris Lane
Laura E. Matthew
Pablo García Loaeza
Rolena Adorno

## Titles in Print